FERTILITY DIET RECIPES COOKBOOK FOR WOMEN

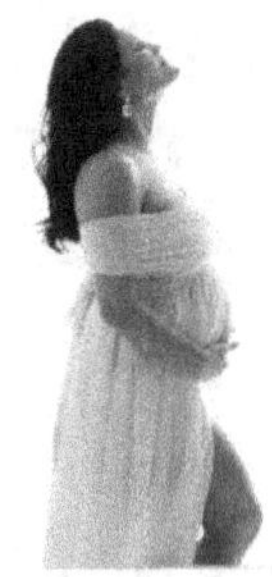

EASY HEALTHY AND DELICIOUS RECIPES TO IMPROVE YOUR EGG QUALITY AND YOUR FERTILITY

TRACY R. LEROY

Copyright page

Copyright Page © 2024

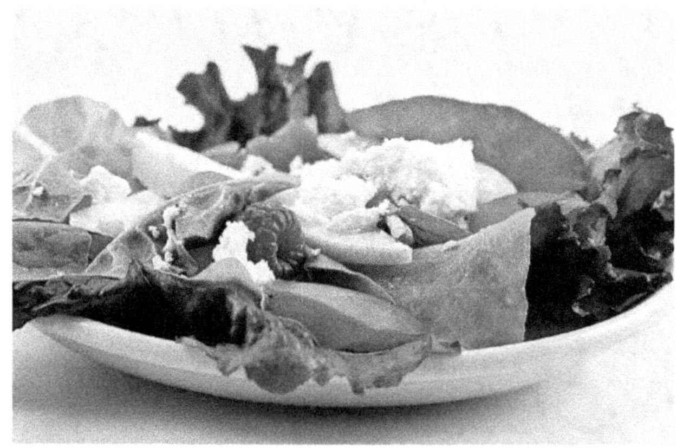

TABLE OF CONTENTS

INTRODUCTION 5

How This Cookbook Can Support Your Journey to Parenthood 7

Chapter 1: 11

Foundations of Fertility Nutrition 11

Tips for Creating a Fertility-Friendly Meal Plan 15

Chapter 2 19

MEAL PLANNING AND PREPARING FOR CONCEPTION
.... 19

14-DAY MEAL PLAN 21

Day 1: 21

Day 2: 22

Day 3: 22

Day 4 23

Day 5: 23

Day 6: 24

Day 7: 24

Day 8: 25

Day 9: 25

Day 10: 26

Day 11: 26

Day 12: 27

Day 13: 27

Day 14: 28

Chapter 3 29

BREAKFAST RECIPES 29

Chapter 4 43

LUNCH RECIPES 43

Chapter 5 63

DINNER 63

Chapter 6 83

SNACKS AND TREATS 83

Chapter 7 95

BEVERAGES 95

Chapter 8 107

LIFESTYLE PRACTICES FOR FERTILITY 107

Incorporating Exercise into Your Routine 107

What are the benefits of physical activities for those who want to get pregnant? 112

The Role of Sleep in Fertility 116

Stress Management Techniques for Both Partners 119

Chapter 9 123

BONUS (FREE 15 SMOOTHIES) 123

Conclusion 135

INTRODUCTION

Sarah felt like her dreams were melting like ice cream on a summer day. Months of trying for a baby, endless doctor visits, and still, her womb remained empty. She and her husband, Tom, my brother, were heartbroken. One day, while searching through an online bookstore, I stumbled upon a bright yellow book, a fertile diet cookbook.

Checking through the pages filled with dishes like "Sunshine Scramble" and "Rainbow Veggie Stir-Fry," I felt a flicker of hope that this could be their chance. This wasn't a boring diet book; it was a burst of deliciousness with a side of fertility boost. Convinced, I bought the book together with 4 other books. I read it and saw how it would be of help to my brother and his wife. I gave it to them after I went and read through it.

Their kitchen became a laboratory of love. They whipped up salmon scrambles bursting with omega-3s, built towers of leafy green salads, and simmered stews brimming with folate. Each meal was a tiny adventure, a playful experiment in making their bodies stronger, healthier, and maybe, just maybe, baby-ready.

But the "Yummy Tummy" meals became their secret weapon, not just nourishing their bodies but also feeding their hope. When I visit them in the summer, they held hands over steaming bowls of lentil soup, their laughter echoing off the walls. Each bite was a reminder that they were in this together, fueling their dream with vibrant vegetables and hearty grains.

And then, one unexpected morning, their world changed. A faint pink line on the pregnancy test, so bright and bold against the white it seemed to glow. Sarah and Tom held each other, tears finally flowing freely, this time with unbridled joy. Their "Yummy Tummy" journey had led them to the most delicious miracle of all - a tiny heartbeat pulsing inside Sarah.

Their son, Oliver, became a walking testament to the power of good food and unwavering hope. As they watched him grow, strong and healthy, Sarah knew they weren't just parents, they were culinary warriors. They'd conquered their fears with every bite, proving that sometimes, the sweetest victory comes in the form of a yellow cookbook and a whole lot of love.

So, to all the hopeful hearts on the fertility journey, take it from Sarah and Tom: grab this cookbook, whip up some "Yummy Tummy" magic, and never give up on the delicious dream of creating a family. You might just find that the key to unlocking your happy ending lies right there, on a plate, waiting to be enjoyed.

After this miraculous turnaround, I decided to write a fertility diet cookbook filtering every unnecessary piece of information and include every detail concerning the diet and recipes that made parents.

How This Cookbook Can Support Your Journey to Parenthood

The importance of a fertility diet cookbook lies in its potential to provide guidance and support for individuals or couples who are actively trying to conceive. Here are some key aspects of the importance of this fertility diet cookbook:

- **Nutritional Support for Reproductive Health**:

This fertility diet cookbook is designed to include foods that are rich in nutrients essential for reproductive health. Nutrients such as folate, iron, zinc, and antioxidants play crucial roles in fertility for both men and women.

- **Hormonal Balance**:

  Certain foods can contribute to hormonal balance, which is essential for regular menstrual cycles in women and overall reproductive function in both genders. This cookbook includes ingredients that support the production and regulation of reproductive hormones.

- **Reduction of Harmful Substances**

This fertility diet cookbook emphasizes the importance of avoiding or minimizing certain substances that can negatively impact fertility, such as excessive caffeine, alcohol, and processed foods. This can contribute to a healthier environment for conception.

- **Weight Management**

Maintaining a healthy weight is vital for fertility. You are provided with recipes that support healthy weight management, as both underweight and overweight conditions can affect fertility.

- **Blood Sugar Regulation**

Stable blood sugar levels are important for overall health and fertility. This cookbook focus on incorporating complex carbohydrates and foods that help regulate blood sugar.

- **Lifestyle Factors**

Beyond nutrition, this fertility diet cookbook addresses lifestyle factors such as regular exercise, stress management, and adequate sleep. These factors contribute to overall well-being and can influence fertility.

BONUS; FREE 15 SMOOTHIES INSIDE THIS BOOK.

GRAB A COPY NOW.

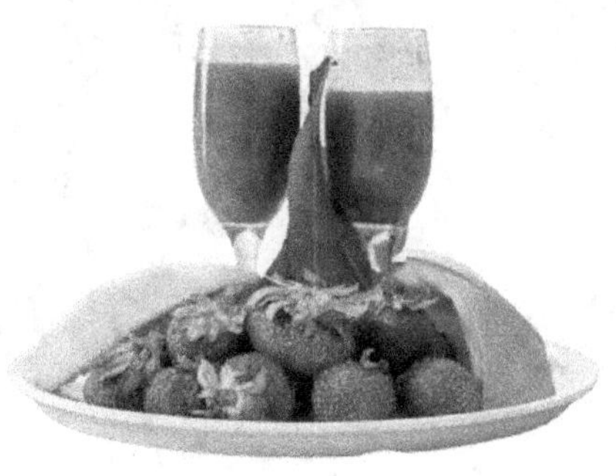

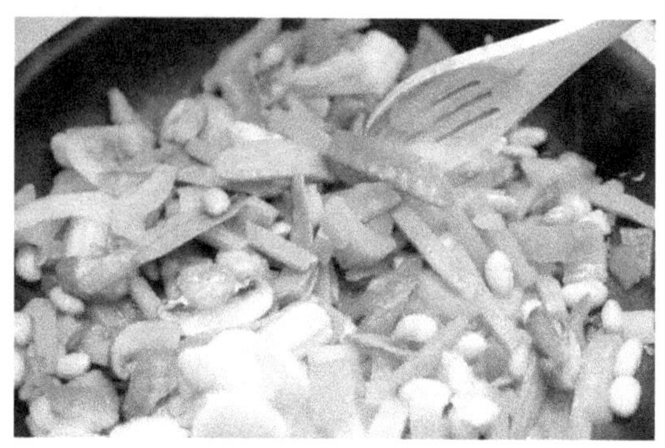

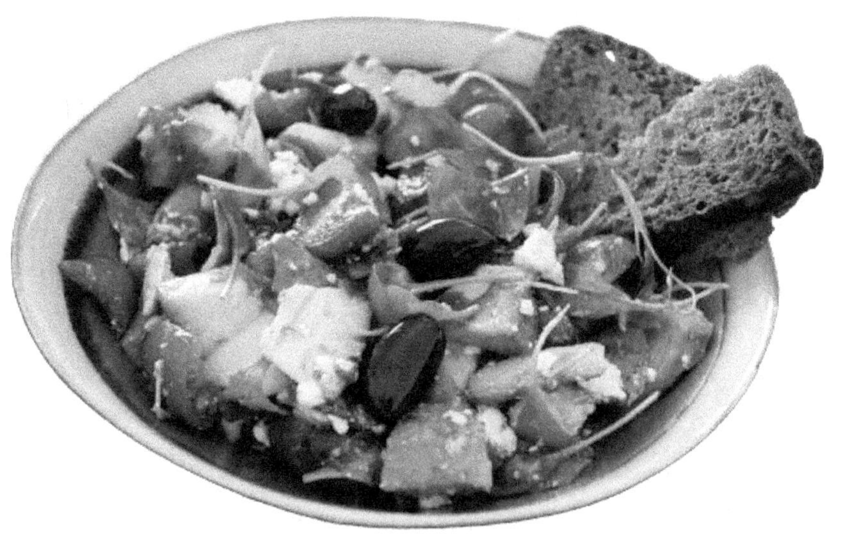

Chapter 1:

Foundations of Fertility Nutrition

However, it is estimated that there is a high percentage of unknown cases, as not everyone seeks medical help.

Considering having a child is a big step in a couple's life. Planning a pregnancy is extremely important, both to guarantee the health of the baby and the mother, and to ensure that the conditions are in place for the couple to conceive without problems.

Infertility is more common than we think

Before talking about the influence of nutrition on fertility, it is worth knowing more about this difficulty or inability to reproduce that affects many people.

According to the World Health Organization (2005), 8 to 15% of couples face some setback in being able to reproduce. In certain parts of the world, this percentage reaches close to 30%, a surprising rate.

Infertility, whether momentary or permanent, can be caused by numerous reasons, such as ovulatory dysfunction, polycystic ovary syndrome, endometriosis, thyroid disorders, stress, sedentary lifestyle or nutritional problems.

Nutrition and fertility are connected, in fact, nutrition is important, also to keep eggs and sperm in good health.

Numerous studies, however, have shown that introducing certain foods into our diet and following certain dietary guidelines can improve ovulation, reduce inflammatory states and reduce the possibility of spontaneous abortions and in males improve the seminal profile.

Our diet plays an important role in keeping our reproductive system healthy and efficient: the substances to "produce" hormones are taken in with food just as many foods are rich in antioxidants which protect oocytes and spermatozoa from free radicals.

At the same time, there are foods and food-related chemicals that can damage your fertility and that you need to know about and avoid.

It's not just a "healthy" diet, but a way of eating that takes your specific problems into account. There is a lot of scientific evidence that highlights how specific foods help or worsen specific clinical situations.

Nutrition is vital for the proper functioning of our body. It has been known to everyone for a long time now. On the other hand, if it is not healthy and balanced it can cause numerous health problems: obesity, cardiovascular diseases, diabetes, etc. The aspect that is often overlooked, or rather underestimated, is its effect on the reproductive system. Well yes, there is a close link between nutrition and infertility.

At a nutritional level, in addition to correcting any dietary errors, it is important to understand if there is any nutritional imbalance, with iron, folic acid, vitamin B12, vitamin D, iodine and calcium being some of the most relevant nutrients. Ensuring a good nutritional status is crucial to ensuring the good development of processes inherent to pregnancy (e.g.: formation and implantation of the placenta, cell differentiation, fetal growth and correct closure of the neural tube).

In terms of diet, it must be varied and healthy, with adequate nutrient intake, similar to the recommendations for the general population. You should adopt a dietary pattern based on starchy foods (choosing whole grain varieties or potatoes with the skin when you can). It should also include lots of fruits and vegetables, moderate amounts of meat, fish and/or other sources of protein (such as eggs and legumes), as well as moderate amounts of dairy products (such as milk, yogurt or cheese). Foods and drinks high in fat and sugar should be consumed in limited quantities.

Nutrition, how it affects fertility

Nutrition affects the fertility of both men and women and is one of the aspects that can easily be changed in order to be able to conceive a child.

To confirm everything, numerous scientific studies have been carried out over time which has highlighted the following:

- Women with an unbalanced diet rich in fats and carbohydrates take longer to remain pregnant, the same happens if they eat little fish
- Saturated fats are the enemy of sperm production
- Sugary drinks such as industrial fruit juices (but also energy and carbonated drinks) have been linked to lower male and female fertility.
- Deficiencies of some vitamins can promote infertility (particularly folates).
- Excessive alcohol consumption has a direct impact on the production of hormones and can therefore complicate ovulation and worsen the production of sperm in quality and quantity.

Tips for Creating a Fertility-Friendly Meal Plan

Creating a fertility-friendly meal plan involves incorporating nutrient-dense foods that support reproductive health. Here are some tips to consider when developing a meal plan to enhance fertility:

- **Include a Variety of Nutrient-Rich Foods**

Ensure your meal plan includes a variety of fruits, vegetables, whole grains, lean proteins, and healthy fats to provide a broad range of essential nutrients. There will be a 14-Day Meal plan in this book to guide you.

Opt for colorful fruits and vegetables, as different colors often indicate various antioxidants and phytochemicals beneficial for reproductive health.

- **Prioritize Healthy Fats**

Avocados, almonds, seeds, and olive oil are all good sources of healthful fats. These fats are important for hormone production and overall reproductive function.

- **Emphasize Plant-Based Proteins**

Choose plant-based protein sources like beans, lentils, quinoa, and tofu. Plant-based proteins can provide essential amino acids without the saturated fats found in some animal products.

- **Incorporate Folate-Rich Foods**

Folate is crucial for fetal development, so include foods rich in folate, such as leafy green vegetables, legumes, and fortified grains.

- **Prioritize Iron-Rich Foods**

Lean meats, chicken, fish, beans, and fortified grains are good sources of iron, which is necessary for good health. Adequate iron levels are important for fertility.

- **Include Omega-3 Fatty Acids**

Include foods high in omega-3 fatty acids, such as walnuts, chia seeds, flaxseeds, and fatty fish (mackerel, salmon). Omega-3s have anti-inflammatory properties that may benefit fertility.

- **Choose Whole Grains**

Opt for whole grains like brown rice, quinoa, and whole wheat, which provide fiber and nutrients. Whole grains can help regulate blood sugar levels, supporting reproductive health.

- **Limit Processed Foods and Added Sugars**

Minimize the intake of processed foods and foods high in added sugars. These can negatively impact hormonal balance and overall health.

- **Stay Hydrated**

Adequate hydration is important for overall health and can support fertility. Water is the perfect beverage throughout the day.

- **Moderate Caffeine and Alcohol Intake**

Limit caffeine intake and consider choosing decaffeinated options. Moderate alcohol consumption is generally recommended, but it's essential to consult with healthcare professionals regarding specific recommendations.

- **Consider Supplements**

Consult with healthcare professionals about appropriate supplements, such as folic acid, vitamin D, and omega-3 fatty acids, to complement your meal plan.

- **Balance Portion Sizes**

Keep an eye on portion amounts to stay within a healthy weight range.. Both underweight and overweight conditions can impact fertility.

Chapter 2

MEAL PLANNING AND PREPARING FOR CONCEPTION

Meal planning for a fertility diet cookbook for couples involves strategically selecting and organizing meals to support reproductive health. Proper management of a fertility-focused meal plan offers several benefits:

1. Balanced Nutrient Intake:

Benefit: Ensures that both partners receive a well-rounded mix of essential nutrients crucial for reproductive health.

Explanation: A balanced diet rich in vitamins, minerals, antioxidants, and other nutrients supports hormonal balance, egg and sperm development, and overall reproductive function.

2. Stable Blood Sugar Levels:

Benefit: Helps maintain stable insulin levels, reducing the risk of insulin resistance and promoting hormonal balance.

Explanation: Stable blood sugar levels support fertility by preventing disruptions in hormonal regulation, which is crucial for menstrual cycle regularity and optimal reproductive function.

3. Healthy Weight Management:

Benefit: Supports achieving and maintaining a healthy weight, which is essential for fertility.

Explanation: Both underweight and overweight conditions can negatively impact fertility. Proper meal planning helps manage calorie intake, ensuring that the body receives the nutrients it needs without excess or deficiency, promoting a healthy weight range.

4. Reduction of Inflammatory Foods:

Benefit: Minimizes the consumption of inflammatory foods that can contribute to reproductive issues.

Explanation: Certain foods may trigger inflammation, which can affect reproductive organs and disrupt hormonal balance. A well-planned fertility diet cookbook emphasizes anti-inflammatory foods, such as fruits, vegetables, and omega-3 fatty acids, while minimizing processed and inflammatory foods.

14-DAY MEAL PLAN

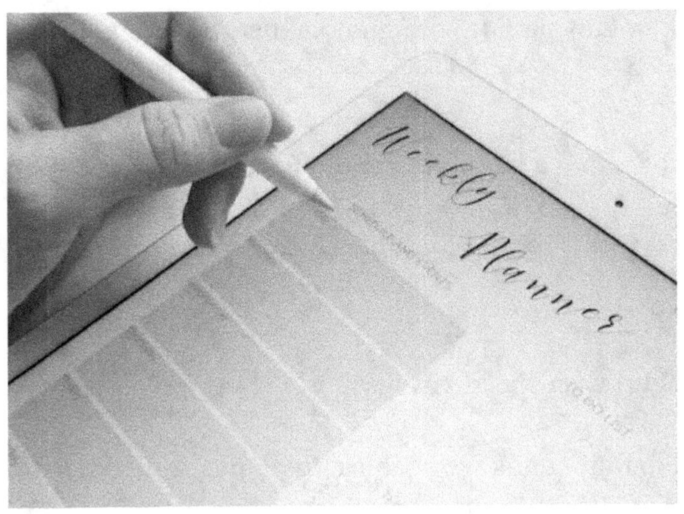

Day 1:

Breakfast: Berry Smoothie (mixed berries, banana, Greek yogurt, chia seeds, almond milk)

Snack: Handful of almonds and an apple

Lunch: Grilled chicken salad with spinach, avocado, cherry tomatoes, and olive oil dressing

Snack: Carrot and cucumber sticks with hummus

Dinner: Baked salmon, quinoa, steamed broccoli, and a side of mixed berries

Day 2:

Breakfast: Greek yogurt parfait with granola, berries, and a drizzle of honey

Snack: Orange slices and a handful of walnuts

Lunch: Lentil soup with whole-grain roll and a side of mixed greens

Snack: Greek yogurt with sliced kiwi

Dinner: Stir-fried tofu withs vegetables (bell peppers, broccoli, carrots) and brown rice

Day 3:

Breakfast: Spinach and feta omelet with whole-grain toast

Snack: Banana and a handful of almonds

Lunch: Quinoa salad with chickpeas, cucumber, tomatoes, and lemon-tahini dressing

Snack: Cottage cheese with pineapple chunks

Dinner: Grilled shrimp, sweet potato wedges, sautéed kale, and a side of mixed berries

Day 4:

Breakfast: Mango and banana smoothie with spinach, Greek yogurt, and almond milk

Snack: Mixed berries and a small handful of pistachios

Lunch: Turkey and avocado wrap with whole-grain tortilla and a side of carrot sticks

Snack: Greek yogurt with sliced strawberries

Dinner: Baked cod fillet, quinoa, roasted Brussels sprouts, and a side of watermelon cubes

Day 5:

Breakfast: Chia seed pudding with coconut milk, topped with sliced peaches and almonds

Snack: Apple slices with almond butter

Lunch: Spinach and strawberry salad with grilled chicken, feta cheese, and balsamic vinaigrette

Snack: Carrot and celery sticks with hummus

Dinner: Eggplant and chickpea curry with brown rice

Day 6:

Breakfast: Blueberry and banana smoothie with spinach, chia seeds, and almond milk

Snack: Handful of mixed nuts and a pear

Lunch: Quinoa-stuffed bell peppers with black beans, corn, and salsa

Snack: Cottage cheese with pineapple chunks

Dinner: Grilled chicken breast, sweet potato mash, steamed asparagus, and a side of mixed berries

Day 7:

Breakfast: Greek yogurt parfait with granola, mango slices, and a drizzle of honey

Snack: Orange slices and a handful of walnuts

Lunch: Lentil and vegetable stir-fry with brown rice

Snack: Banana and a small handful of pistachios

Dinner: Baked salmon, quinoa, roasted Brussels sprouts, and a side of watermelon cubes

Day 8:

Breakfast: Spinach and mushroom omelet with whole-grain toast

Snack: Apple slices with almond butter

Lunch: Turkey and avocado wrap with whole-grain tortilla and a side of carrot sticks

Snack: Carrot and celery sticks with hummus

Dinner: Stir-fried tofu with broccoli, bell peppers, and brown rice

Day 9:

Breakfast: Chia seed pudding with coconut milk, topped with sliced strawberries and almonds

Snack: Mixed berries and a handful of cashews

Lunch: Quinoa salad with chickpeas, cucumber, tomatoes, and lemon-tahini dressing

Snack: Greek yogurt with sliced kiwi

Dinner: Eggplant and chickpea curry with quinoa

Day 10:

Breakfast: Mango and banana smoothie with spinach, Greek yogurt, and almond milk

Snack: Handful of mixed nuts and an apple

Lunch: Grilled shrimp, quinoa, sautéed kale, and a side of mixed berries

Snack: Carrot and cucumber sticks with hummus

Dinner: Baked cod fillet, sweet potato wedges, steamed broccoli, and a side of watermelon cubes

Day 11:

Breakfast: Blueberry and banana smoothie with kale, chia seeds, and coconut water

Snack: Orange slices and a handful of walnuts

Lunch: Lentil soup with whole-grain roll and a side of mixed greens

Snack: Greek yogurt with sliced strawberries

Dinner: Spinach and feta stuffed chicken breast, quinoa, roasted Brussels sprouts, and a side of mixed berries

Day 12:

Breakfast: Greek yogurt parfait with granola, peach slices, and a drizzle of honey

Snack: Banana and a small handful of pistachios

Lunch: Turkey and avocado salad with mixed greens, cherry tomatoes, and balsamic vinaigrette

Snack: Cottage cheese with pineapple chunks

Dinner: Stir-fried tofu with vegetables (bell peppers, broccoli, carrots) and brown rice

Day 13:

Breakfast: Spinach and mushroom omelet with whole-grain toast

Snack: Apple slices with almond butter

Lunch: Quinoa-stuffed bell peppers with black beans, corn, and salsa

Snack: Carrot and celery sticks with hummus

Dinner: Grilled chicken breast, sweet potato mash, steamed asparagus, and a side of mixed berries

Day 14:

Breakfast: Chia seed pudding with coconut milk, topped with sliced strawberries and almonds

Snack: Mixed berries and a handful of cashews

Lunch: Lentil and vegetable stir-fry with brown rice

Snack: Greek yogurt with sliced kiwi

Dinner: Eggplant and chickpea curry with quinoa

Chapter 3

BREAKFAST RECIPES

1. Berry Nut Smoothie

<u>Prep Time</u>: 10 minutes

<u>Ingredients</u>:

1 cup mixed berries (blueberries, strawberries, raspberries)

1 banana

1/4 cup Greek yogurt

2 tablespoons chia seeds

1/4 cup almonds (sliced)

1 tablespoon honey

<u>Instructions</u>:

Blend together the berries, banana, and Greek yoghurt until smooth.

Pour into a bowl and top with chia seeds, sliced almonds, and a drizzle of honey.

2. Spinach and Feta Omelette

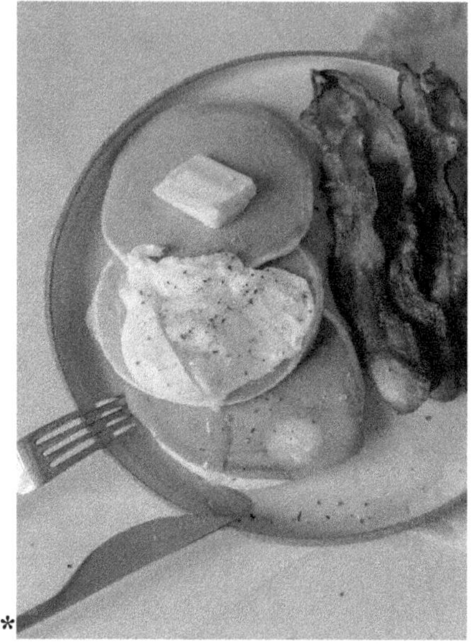

Prep Time: 15 minutes

Ingredients:

3 eggs

1 cup fresh spinach (chopped)

1/4 cup feta cheese (crumbled)

1 tablespoon olive oil

Salt and pepper to taste

Description: Packed with folate and protein, this omelette is perfect for a fertility diet.

Instructions:

Add salt and pepper to the eggs as you whisk them.

Sauté spinach in olive oil until wilted.

Pour eggs over spinach, add feta, cook until set, and fold.

3. Quinoa Breakfast Bowl

Prep Time: 20 minutes

Ingredients:

1 cup cooked quinoa

1/2 cup mixed berries

1/4 cup nuts (walnuts or almonds)

1 tablespoon honey

1/2 cup Greek yogurt

Description: A nutrient-packed bowl rich in protein, fiber, and antioxidants.

Instructions:

Mix cooked quinoa with Greek yogurt.

Garnish with nuts and berries and pour honey over the top.

4. Avocado Toast with Poached Egg

Prep Time: 15 minutes

Ingredients:

1 slice whole-grain bread

1/2 avocado (mashed)

1 egg (poached)

Salt, pepper, and red pepper flakes to taste

Description: Avocado provides healthy fats, while the egg adds protein and vitamins.

Instructions:

Toast bread, spread mashed avocado.

Top with a poached egg and season to taste.

5. Chia Seed Pudding Parfait

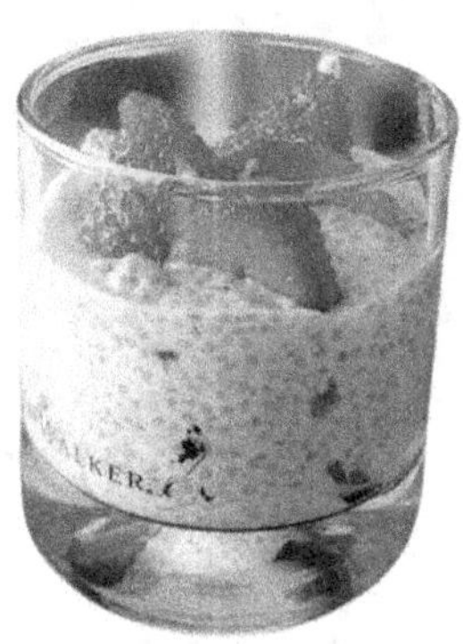

<u>Prep Time</u>: 5 minutes (plus chilling time)

<u>Ingredients</u>:

2 tablespoons chia seeds

1 cup almond milk

1/2 cup granola

1/2 cup mixed berries

<u>Description</u>: Chia seeds are a great source of omega-3 fatty acids and fiber.

Mix chia seeds with almond milk and refrigerate until it thickens.

Layer chia pudding with granola and berries.

6. Sweet Potato Hash

Prep Time: 25 minutes

Ingredients:

1 sweet potato (grated)

1/2 onion (chopped)

1 bell pepper (chopped)

2 eggs

2 tablespoons olive oil

Salt and pepper to taste

Description: Packed with beta-carotene, fiber, and protein.

Instructions:

Sauté sweet potato, onion, and bell pepper in olive oil.

Create wells in the mixture, crack eggs into them, and cook until eggs are done.

7. Fruit and Nut Yogurt Parfait

<u>Prep Time</u>: 10 minutes

<u>Ingredients</u>:

1 cup Greek yogurt

1/2 cup mixed berries

1/4 cup nuts (pistachios or almonds)

1 tablespoon honey

<u>Description</u>: A protein-packed and vitamin-rich parfait.

<u>Instructions</u>:

Layer Greek yogurt with berries and nuts.

Drizzle with honey before serving.

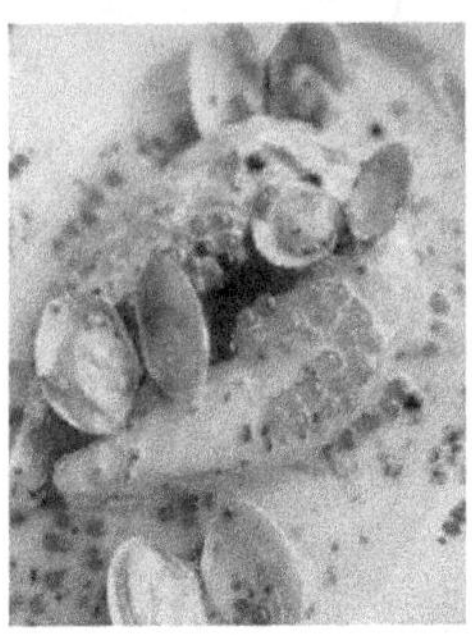

8. Salmon and Asparagus Frittata

<u>Prep Time</u>: 30 minutes

<u>Ingredients</u>:

4 eggs

1/2 cup smoked salmon (flaked)

1/2 cup asparagus (chopped)

1/4 cup feta cheese (crumbled)

Salt and pepper to taste

<u>Description</u>: Omega-3 fatty acids from salmon and fertility-boosting nutrients from asparagus.

<u>Instructions</u>:

Whisk eggs, add salmon, asparagus, feta, salt, and pepper.

Bake until set.

9. Cottage Cheese Pancakes

Prep Time: 15 minutes

Ingredients:

1 cup cottage cheese

2 eggs

1/2 cup oats (blended into flour)

1 teaspoon vanilla extract

1/2 cup mixed berries

Description: High in protein and calcium.

Instructions:

Blend cottage cheese, eggs, oat flour, and vanilla.

Cook pancakes and top with berries.

10. Blueberry Almond Overnight Oats

Prep Time: 5 minutes (plus overnight chilling)

Ingredients:

1/2 cup rolled oats

1/2 cup almond milk

1/4 cup blueberries

1 tablespoon almond butter

1 teaspoon chia seeds

<u>Description</u>: A make-ahead, fiber-rich breakfast.

<u>Instructions</u>:

Mix oats with almond milk and refrigerate overnight.

Top with blueberries, almond butter, and chia seeds before serving.

11. Pomegranate and Walnut Quinoa Porridge

<u>Prep Time</u>: 20 minutes

<u>Ingredients</u>:

1/2 cup quinoa (rinsed)

1 cup almond milk

1/4 cup pomegranate seeds

2 tablespoons chopped walnuts

1 tablespoon maple syrup

Description: Quinoa provides essential amino acids, while pomegranate seeds add antioxidants.

Instructions:

Cook quinoa in almond milk, top with pomegranate seeds, walnuts, and maple syrup.

12. Egg and Veggie Breakfast Burrito

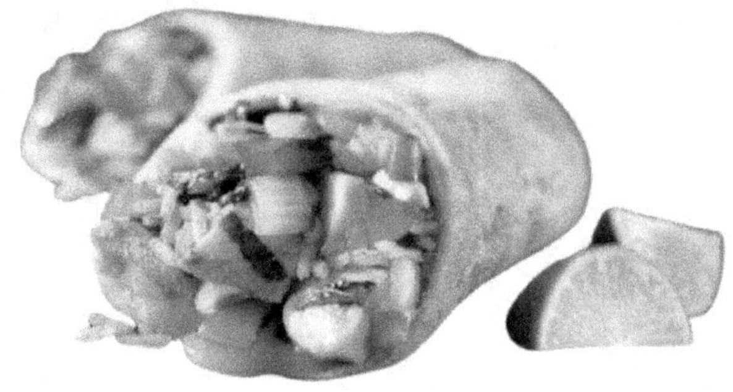

Prep Time: 20 minutes

Ingredients:

2 eggs (scrambled)

1 whole-grain tortilla

1/2 cup black beans (cooked)

1/4 cup salsa

1/4 avocado (sliced)

Description: A hearty breakfast rich in protein and fiber.

Instructions:

Fill tortilla with scrambled eggs, black beans, salsa, and avocado.

13. Mango Spinach Green Smoothie

Prep Time: 10 minutes

Ingredients:

1 cup spinach

1/2 cup mango (frozen)

1/2 banana

1/2 cup coconut water

1 tablespoon chia seeds

Description: A vitamin-packed smoothie for a refreshing start.

Instructions:

Blend spinach, mango, banana, coconut water, and chia seeds until smooth.

14. Whole Grain Waffles with Berries

Prep Time: 15 minutes

Ingredients:

1 cup whole-grain waffle mix

1 egg

1 cup mixed berries

1 tablespoon maple syrup

Description: Whole grains provide essential nutrients for fertility.

Instructions:

Prepare waffle mix with egg, cook, and top with berries and maple syrup.

15. Protein-Packed Peanut Butter Smoothie

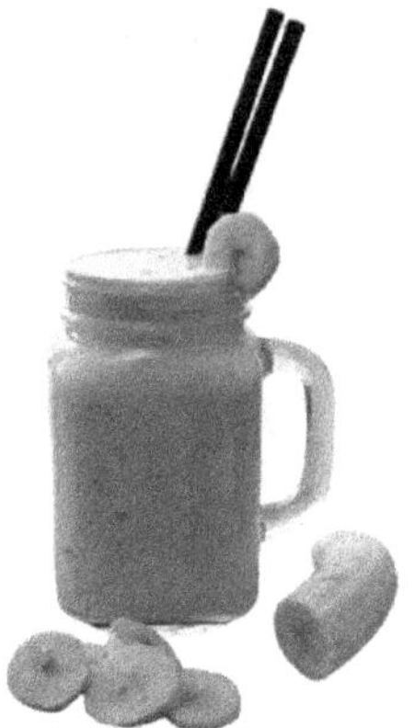

<u>Prep Time</u>: 10 minutes

<u>Ingredients</u>:

1 banana

2 tablespoons peanut butter

1 scoop protein powder

1 cup almond milk

1/2 teaspoon cinnamon

<u>Description</u>: A protein-rich smoothie with healthy fats.

<u>Instructions</u>:

Blend banana, peanut butter, protein powder, almond milk, and cinnamon until smooth.

Chapter 4

LUNCH RECIPES

1. Quinoa Salad with Avocado and Pomegranate

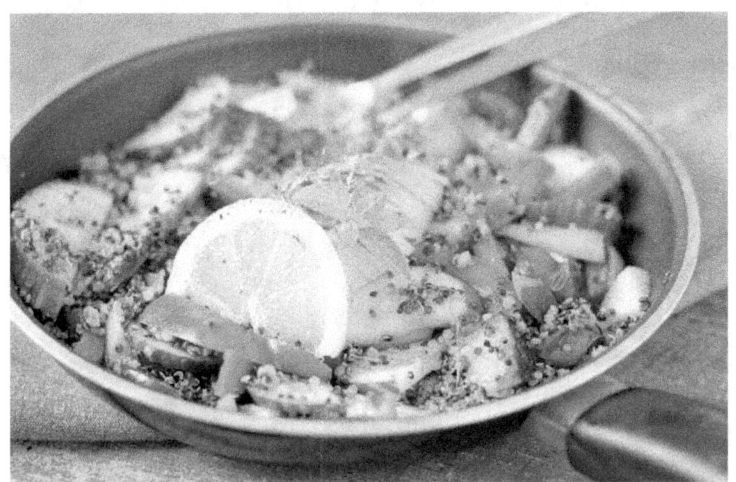

Prep Time: 20 minutes

Ingredients:

1 cup cooked quinoa

1 ripe avocado, diced

1/2 cup pomegranate seeds

1/4 cup chopped fresh cilantro

2 tablespoons extra-virgin olive oil

Juice of 1 lemon

Salt and pepper to taste

Description: A refreshing and nutrient-packed salad rich in healthy fats and antioxidants.

Instructions:

In a large bowl, combine quinoa, diced avocado, pomegranate seeds, and cilantro.

In a small bowl, whisk together olive oil, lemon juice, salt, and pepper.

After adding the dressing to the salad, gently toss to mix it in.

2. Grilled Salmon with Asparagus

Prep Time: 25 minutes

Ingredients:

2 salmon fillets

1 bunch asparagus, trimmed

2 tablespoons olive oil

1 teaspoon lemon zest

1 teaspoon chopped fresh dill

Salt and pepper to taste

<u>Description</u>: A protein-rich dish with omega-3 fatty acids and essential nutrients.

Instructions:

Preheat the grill. Brush salmon fillets and asparagus with olive oil.

Season salmon with lemon zest, dill, salt, and pepper.

Grill salmon for 4-5 minutes per side and asparagus for 3-4 minutes until tender.

2. Lentil and Vegetable Stew

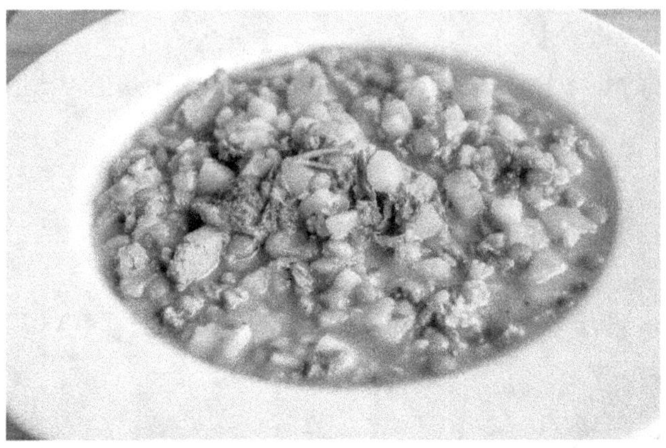

<u>Prep Time</u>: 30 minutes

<u>Ingredients</u>:

1 cup dry green lentils, rinsed

2 carrots, chopped

1 zucchini, diced

1 onion, finely chopped

3 cloves garlic, minced

1 can diced tomatoes

4 cups vegetable broth

1 teaspoon cumin

1 teaspoon paprika

Salt and pepper to taste

<u>Description</u>: A hearty stew loaded with fertility-friendly lentils and colorful vegetables.

<u>Instructions</u>:

Sauté the onion and garlic in a big saucepan until they become aromatic.

Add carrots, zucchini, lentils, diced tomatoes, vegetable broth, cumin, paprika, salt, and pepper.

Lentils should simmer for 25 to 30 minutes to become soft.

4. Sweet Potato and Chickpea Buddha Bowl

Prep Time: 25 minutes

Ingredients:

2 sweet potatoes, cubed

1 can chickpeas, rinsed and drained

1 cup quinoa, cooked

1 cup kale, chopped

2 tablespoons tahini

1 tablespoon lemon juice

1 teaspoon ground cumin

Salt and pepper to taste

Description: A nutrient-packed bowl with fertility-boosting ingredients.

<u>Instructions</u>:

Roast sweet potatoes and chickpeas in olive oil until golden brown.

In a bowl, assemble quinoa, roasted sweet potatoes, chickpeas, and kale.

Drizzle with a dressing made from tahini, lemon juice, cumin, salt, and pepper.

5. Spinach and Berry Salad with Grilled Chicken

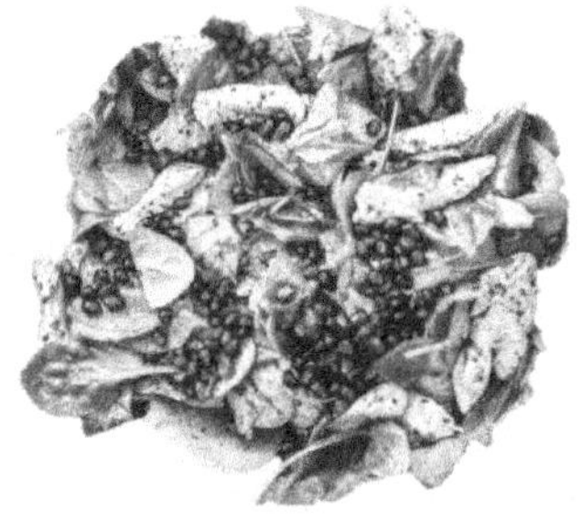

<u>Prep Time</u>: 15 minutes

<u>Ingredients</u>:

2 boneless, skinless chicken breasts

4 cups fresh spinach

1 cup mixed berries (blueberries, strawberries)

1/4 cup feta cheese, crumbled

2 tablespoons balsamic vinaigrette

1 tablespoon olive oil

Salt and pepper to taste

Description: A vibrant salad with antioxidants, iron, and lean protein.

Instructions:

Season chicken with salt and pepper, grill until cooked through, and slice.

In a large bowl, combine spinach, berries, grilled chicken, and feta.

Drizzle with balsamic vinaigrette and olive oil.

6. Shrimp and Vegetable Stir-Fry

Prep Time: 20 minutes

Ingredients:

1 lb shrimp, peeled and deveined

2 cups broccoli florets

1 bell pepper, sliced

1 carrot, julienned

2 tablespoons soy sauce

1 tablespoon honey

1 tablespoon ginger, minced

2 cloves garlic, minced

2 tablespoons sesame oil

Description: A quick and flavorful stir-fry rich in protein and veggies.

Instructions:

In a wok or skillet, heat sesame oil. Add ginger and garlic, stir briefly.

Add shrimp and vegetables, stir-fry until shrimp turn pink and vegetables are tender.

Mix soy sauce and honey, pour over the stir-fry, and toss until coated.

7. Mediterranean Chickpea Salad

Prep Time: 15 minutes

Ingredients:

1 can chickpeas, rinsed and drained

1 cucumber, diced

1 cup cherry tomatoes, halved

1/2 red onion, finely chopped

1/4 cup feta cheese, crumbled

2 tablespoons olive oil

1 tablespoon red wine vinegar

1 teaspoon dried oregano

Salt and pepper to taste

Description: A refreshing and fiber-rich salad with Mediterranean flavors.

Instructions:

In a large bowl, combine chickpeas, cucumber, cherry tomatoes, red onion, and feta.

In a small bowl, whisk together olive oil, red wine vinegar, oregano, salt, and pepper.

Gently mix the salad after adding the dressing.

8. Egg and Spinach Wrap

<u>Prep Time</u>: 15 minutes

<u>Ingredients</u>:

2 whole wheat tortillas

4 eggs, scrambled

2 cups fresh spinach

1 tomato, diced

1/4 cup shredded mozzarella cheese

Salt and pepper to taste

<u>Description</u>: A protein-packed wrap with essential nutrients.

<u>Instructions</u>:

Scramble eggs in a pan, season with salt and pepper.

Place a tortilla on a plate, layer with spinach, scrambled eggs, tomato, and cheese.

Roll into a wrap and secure with a toothpick.

9. Turkey and Quinoa Stuffed Peppers

Prep Time: 40 minutes

Ingredients:

4 bell peppers, halved and seeds removed

1 lb ground turkey

1 cup cooked quinoa

1 cup black beans, drained and rinsed

1 cup corn kernels

1 cup salsa

1 teaspoon cumin

1 teaspoon chili powder

Salt and pepper to taste

<u>Description</u>: Stuffed peppers with lean protein and fiber.

<u>Instructions</u>:

Preheat the oven to 375°F (190°C).

In a skillet, cook ground turkey until browned. Add cooked quinoa, black beans, corn, salsa, cumin, chili powder, salt, and pepper. Mix well.

Fill each bell pepper half with the turkey and quinoa mixture. Bake for 25-30 minutes.

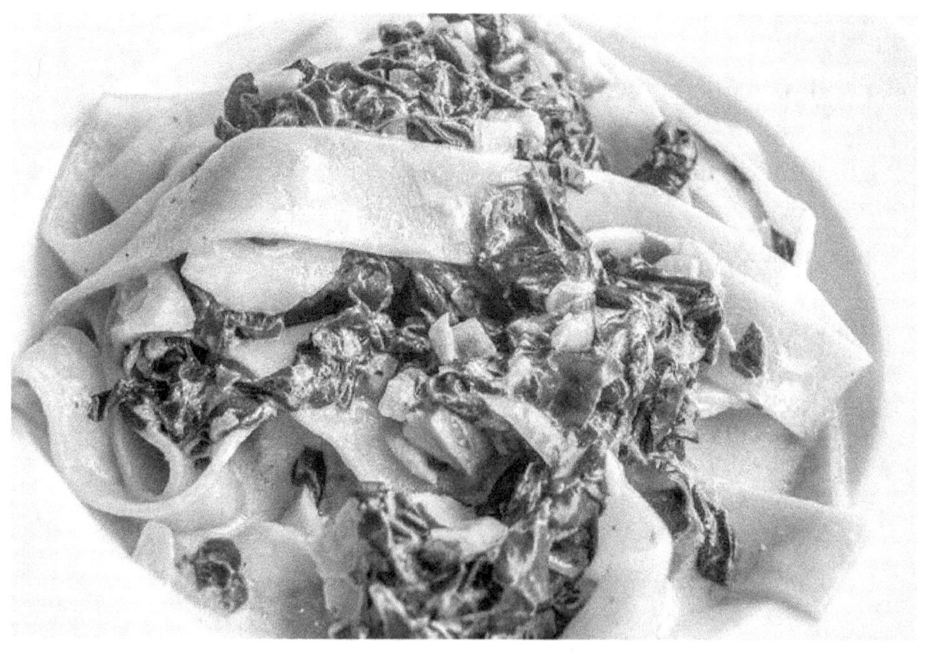

10. Berry and Almond Smoothie Bowl

Prep Time: 10 minutes

Ingredients:

1 cup mixed berries (strawberries, blueberries, raspberries)

1 banana, frozen

1/2 cup almond milk

1/4 cup Greek yogurt

2 tablespoons almond butter

Toppings: sliced almonds, chia seeds, shredded coconut

Description: A nutrient-packed smoothie bowl with antioxidants and healthy fats.

Instructions:

Blend berries, frozen banana, almond milk, Greek yogurt, and almond butter until smooth.

Transfer into a bowl and garnish with shredded coconut, chia seeds, and almond slices.

11. Chicken and Vegetable Brown Rice Bowl

<u>Prep Time</u>: 30 minutes

<u>Ingredients</u>:

1 cup brown rice, cooked

1 lb chicken breast, thinly sliced

2 cups broccoli florets

1 bell pepper, sliced

1 carrot, julienned

2 tablespoons low-sodium soy sauce

1 tablespoon hoisin sauce

1 tablespoon sesame oil

1 teaspoon ginger, minced

2 cloves garlic, minced

<u>Description</u>: A wholesome brown rice bowl with lean protein and veggies.

<u>Instructions</u>:

In a large skillet, heat sesame oil. Add ginger and garlic, stir briefly.

Add chicken and stir-fry until cooked. Add broccoli, bell pepper, and carrot.

Mix soy sauce and hoisin sauce, pour over the chicken and vegetables. Stir until coated.

Serve over cooked brown rice.

12. Tuna and White Bean Salad

<u>Prep Time</u>: 15 minutes

<u>Ingredients</u>:

2 cans tuna, drained

1 can white beans, drained and rinsed

1 cucumber, diced

1 red onion, finely chopped

1/4 cup fresh parsley, chopped

2 tablespoons olive oil

1 tablespoon red wine vinegar

Salt and pepper to taste

<u>Description</u>: A protein-rich salad with omega-3 fatty acids and fiber.

Instructions:

In a large bowl, combine tuna, white beans, cucumber, red onion, and parsley.

In a small bowl, whisk together olive oil, red wine vinegar, salt, and pepper.

Drizzle the salad with the dressing and carefully stir.

13. Veggie and Quinoa Stuffed Acorn Squash

<u>Prep Time</u>: 45 minutes

<u>Ingredients</u>:

2 acorn squash, halved and seeds removed

1 cup quinoa, cooked

1 cup black beans, drained and rinsed

1 cup corn kernels

1 red bell pepper, diced

1/2 cup cilantro, chopped

1 teaspoon cumin

1 teaspoon chili powder

Salt and pepper to taste

Description: Nutrient-dense stuffed acorn squash with quinoa and colorful vegetables.

Instructions:

Preheat the oven to 375°F (190°C).

Place acorn squash halves on a baking sheet. Roast for 25-30 minutes until tender.

In a bowl, mix cooked quinoa, black beans, corn, red bell pepper, cilantro, cumin, chili powder, salt, and pepper.

Stuff each acorn squash half with the quinoa mixture.

14. Mushroom and Spinach Omelette

Prep Time: 15 minutes

Ingredients:

3 eggs, beaten

1 cup spinach, chopped

1/2 cup mushrooms, sliced

1/4 cup feta cheese, crumbled

1 tablespoon olive oil

Salt and pepper to taste

Description: A protein-packed omelette with iron-rich spinach and mushrooms.

Instructions

In a skillet, heat olive oil. Add mushrooms and sauté until golden.

Add chopped spinach and cook until wilted.

Pour beaten eggs over the vegetables. Sprinkle feta cheese, salt, and pepper.

Cook until the edges are set, then fold the omelette in half.

15. Black Bean and Sweet Potato Quesadillas

<u>Prep Time</u>: 30 minutes

<u>Ingredients</u>:

4 whole wheat tortillas

1 can black beans, drained and rinsed

2 sweet potatoes, cooked and mashed

1 cup corn kernels

1 teaspoon cumin

1 teaspoon chili powder

1 cup shredded cheddar cheese

2 tablespoons olive oil

<u>Description</u>: Flavorful quesadillas with black beans, sweet potatoes, and melted cheese.

<u>Instructions</u>:

In a bowl, mix black beans, mashed sweet potatoes, corn, cumin, and chili powder.

Spread the mixture onto half of each tortilla. Sprinkle with cheddar cheese.

Fold the tortillas in half. In a skillet, heat olive oil and cook the quesadillas until golden on both sides.

These recipes are designed to be part of a balanced fertility diet, providing essential nutrients to support reproductive health.

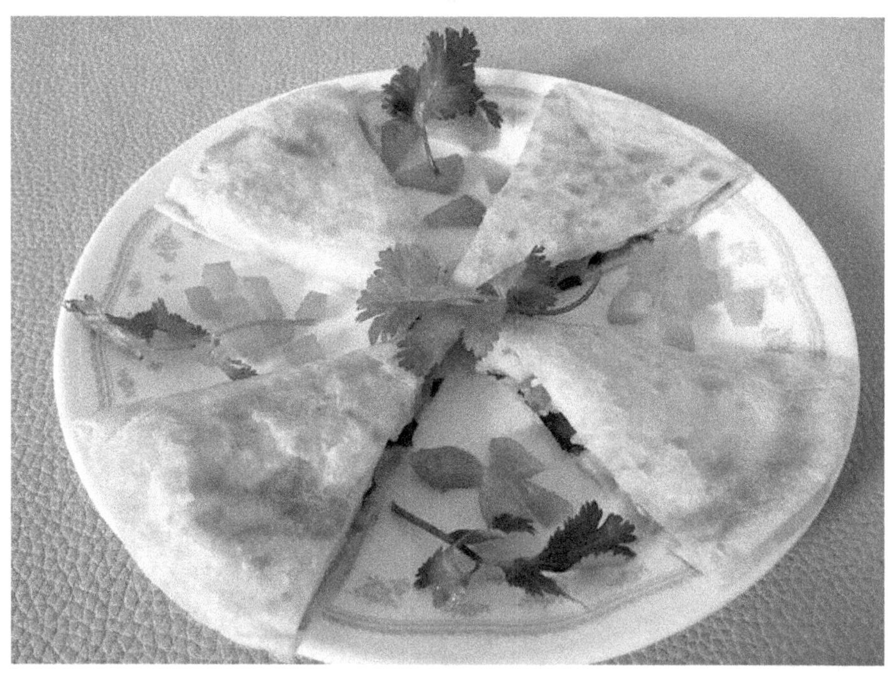

Chapter 5

DINNER

1. Grilled Salmon with Quinoa and Asparagus

Ingredients:

2 salmon fillets

1 cup quinoa

1 bunch asparagus

Olive oil

Lemon juice

Salt and pepper to taste

Preparation:

Cook quinoa according to package instructions.

Season salmon with salt, pepper, and lemon juice. Grill for 5-7 minutes per side.

Roast asparagus with olive oil, salt, and pepper in the oven for 10 minutes.

Serve salmon over a bed of quinoa with asparagus on the side.

<u>Nutritional Value</u>: Rich in Omega-3 fatty acids, protein, and folate.

<u>Prep Time</u>: 30 minutes

2. Lentil and Vegetable Stir-Fry

<u>Ingredients</u>:

1 cup lentils

2 cups broccoli florets

1 bell pepper, thinly sliced

1 carrot, julienned

2 cloves garlic, minced

Soy sauce

Ginger, grated

Olive oil

<u>Preparation</u>:

Cook lentils according to package instructions.

Stir-fry broccoli, bell pepper, carrot, and garlic in olive oil.

Add cooked lentils, soy sauce, and ginger. Cook for an additional 5 minutes.

<u>Nutritional Value</u>: High in protein, fiber, and essential nutrients.

Prep Time:25 minutes

3. Spinach and Chickpea Salad

<u>Ingredients</u>:

2 cups spinach leaves

1 can chickpeas, drained

Cherry tomatoes, halved

Feta cheese

Olive oil

Balsamic vinegar

Salt and pepper to taste

<u>Preparation</u>:

Combine spinach, chickpeas, tomatoes, and feta in a bowl.

Over the salad, drizzle some olive oil and balsamic vinegar.

Season with salt and pepper, toss gently, and serve.

<u>Nutritional Value</u>: Packed with iron, folate, and antioxidants.

<u>Prep Time</u>: 15 minutes

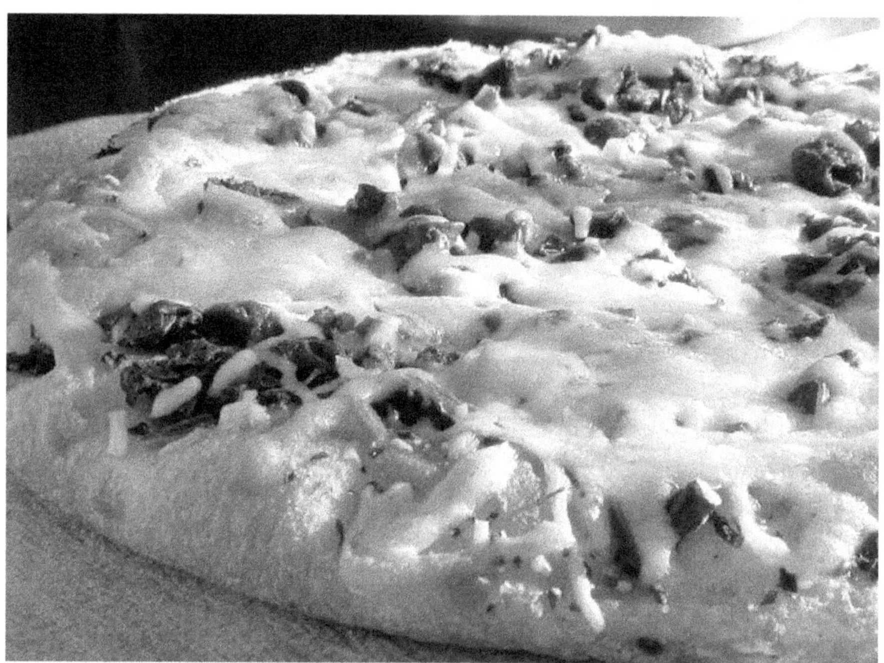

4. Quinoa and Black Bean Stuffed Bell Peppers

<u>Ingredients</u>:

4 bell peppers, halved

1 cup quinoa

1 can black beans, rinsed

Corn kernels

Cumin powder

Tomato sauce

Shredded cheese

Preparation:

Cook quinoa according to package instructions.

Mix quinoa, black beans, corn, cumin, and half of the tomato sauce.

Stuff bell peppers with the mixture, top with the remaining sauce and cheese.

Bake until peppers are tender.

<u>Nutritional Value</u>: Excellent source of protein, fiber, and vitamins.

<u>Prep Time</u>: 40 minutes

5. Sweet Potato and Chickpea Curry

<u>Ingredients</u>:

2 sweet potatoes, diced

1 can chickpeas, drained

1 onion, diced

2 tomatoes, chopped

Coconut milk

Curry powder

Turmeric

Cilantro for garnish

Preparation:

Sauté onion until translucent. Add curry powder and turmeric.

Add sweet potatoes, chickpeas, and tomatoes. Stir well.

Pour in coconut milk and boil until sweet potatoes are cooked.

Garnish with cilantro before serving.

Nutritional Value: High in antioxidants, fiber, and fertility-boosting nutrients.

Prep Time: 35 minutes

6. Shrimp and Vegetable Quinoa Bowl

<u>Ingredients</u>:

1 cup quinoa

1 lb shrimp, peeled and deveined

Broccoli florets

Bell peppers, sliced

Garlic, minced

Soy sauce

Sesame oil

<u>Preparation</u>:

Cook quinoa according to package instructions.

Sauté shrimp, broccoli, bell peppers, and garlic in sesame oil.

Add soy sauce and cook until shrimp are pink and veggies are tender.

Serve over a bed of quinoa.

<u>Nutritional Value:</u> Rich in protein, omega-3 fatty acids, and vitamins.

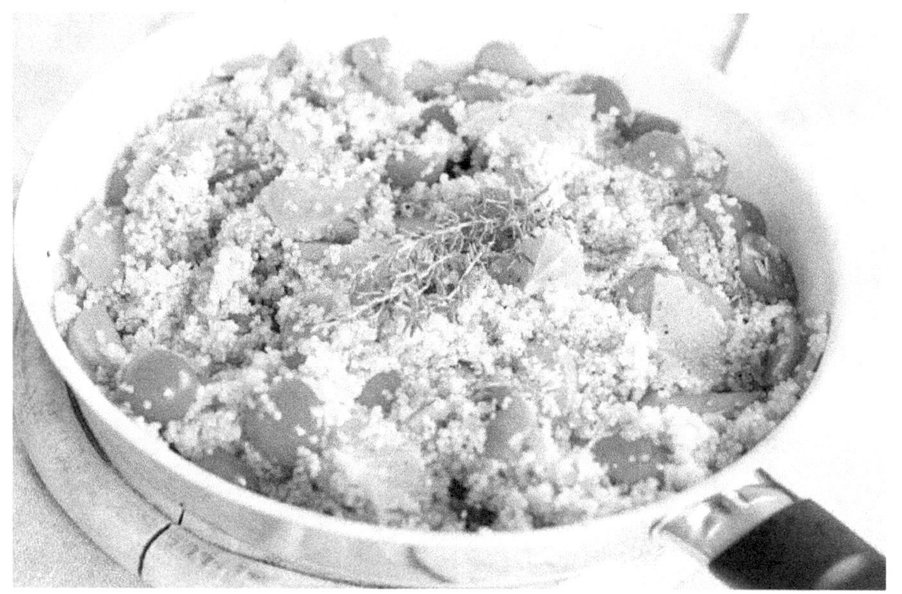

7. Mushroom and Spinach Frittata

Ingredients:

6 eggs

Mushrooms, sliced

Spinach leaves

Feta cheese

Onion, diced

Olive oil

Salt and pepper to taste

<u>Preparation</u>:

In olive oil, sauté onions and mushrooms until they become tender.

Add spinach and cook until wilted.

Whisk eggs, season with salt and pepper, and pour over the veggies.

Crumble feta on top and bake until set.

<u>Nutritional Value</u>: High in protein, iron, and folate.

<u>Prep Time</u>: 30 minutes

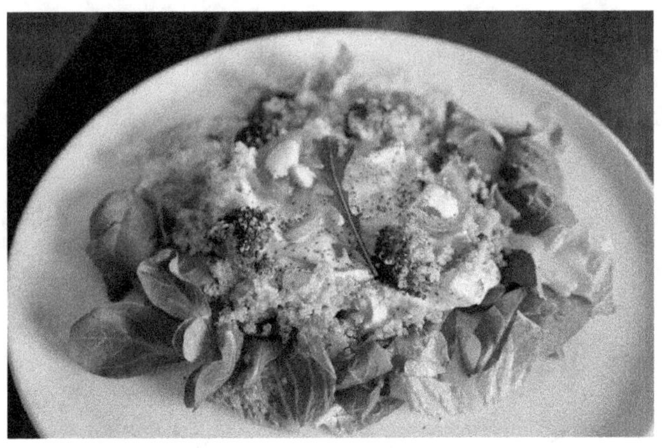

8. Turkey and Quinoa Stuffed Zucchini

Ingredients:

4 zucchinis, halved

1 lb ground turkey

1 cup cooked quinoa

Onion, finely chopped

Tomato sauce

Italian seasoning

Parmesan cheese

Preparation:

Scoop out zucchini centers. Sauté onion and turkey until browned.

Mix cooked quinoa, turkey mixture, and half of the tomato sauce.

Stuff zucchini with the mixture, top with remaining sauce and Parmesan.

Bake until zucchini is tender.

Nutritional Value: Protein-packed and rich in fertility-boosting nutrients.

9. Avocado and Black Bean Salad

Ingredients:

2 avocados, diced

1 can black beans, rinsed

Red onion, finely chopped

Cilantro, chopped

Lime juice

Olive oil

Salt and pepper to taste

Preparation:

Combine avocados, black beans, red onion, and cilantro in a bowl.

Drizzle lime juice and olive oil over the salad.

Season with salt and pepper, toss gently, and serve.

Nutritional Value: Healthy fats, fiber, and fertility-boosting nutrients.

<u>Prep Time</u>: 20 minutes

10. Chicken and Vegetable Skewers

Ingredients:

1 lb chicken breast, cut into chunks

Cherry tomatoes

Bell peppers, cut into squares

Zucchini, sliced

Olive oil

Garlic powder

Paprika

Lemon juice

<u>Preparation</u>:

Thread chicken and vegetables onto skewers.

Mix olive oil, garlic powder, paprika, and lemon juice.

Brush skewers with the mixture and grill until chicken is cooked through.

Nutritional Value: Rich in protein and loaded with several vitamins and minerals.

Prep Time: 30 minutes

11. Quinoa and Vegetable Stuffed Peppers

Ingredients:

4 bell peppers, halved

1 cup quinoa

Mixed vegetables (zucchini, carrots, peas)

Tomato sauce

Italian herbs

Mozzarella cheese

Preparation:

Cook quinoa according to package instructions.

Sauté mixed vegetables in olive oil.

Mix cooked quinoa, vegetables, half of the tomato sauce, and Italian herbs.

Stuff bell peppers, top with the remaining sauce and mozzarella.

Bake until peppers are tender.

<u>Nutritional Value</u>: High in fiber, vitamins, and fertility-boosting nutrients.

<u>Prep Time</u>: 40 minutes

12. Salmon and Broccoli Casserole

<u>Ingredients</u>:

2 salmon fillets, cooked and flaked

2 cups broccoli florets

Brown rice

Greek yogurt

Dijon mustard

Lemon zest

Parmesan cheese

<u>Preparation</u>:

Cook brown rice according to package instructions.

Steam broccoli until tender.

Mix cooked salmon, broccoli, brown rice, Greek yogurt, Dijon mustard, and lemon zest.

Transfer to a baking dish, top with Parmesan, and bake until bubbly.

<u>Nutritional Value</u>: Rich in omega-3 fatty acids, protein, and fertility-boosting nutrients.

<u>Prep Time:</u> 35 minutes

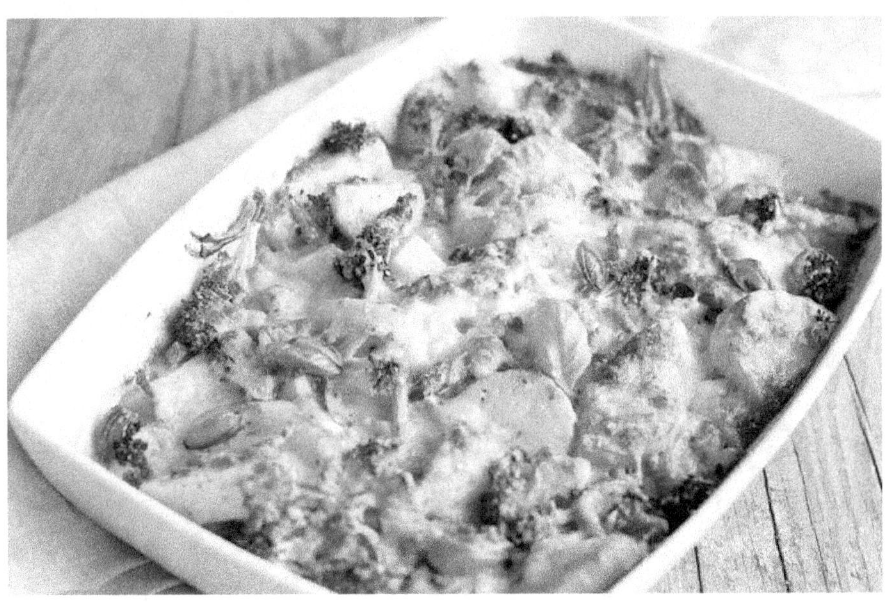

13. Vegetable and Chickpea Quinoa Bowl

Ingredients:

1 cup quinoa

1 can chickpeas, drained

Cherry tomatoes, halved

Cucumber, diced

Red onion, finely chopped

Feta cheese

Olive oil

Lemon juice

Preparation:

Cook quinoa according to package instructions.

Combine quinoa, chickpeas, tomatoes, cucumber, red onion, and feta in a bowl.

Drizzle olive oil and lemon juice over the bowl, toss gently, and serve.

<u>Nutritional Value</u>: High in fiber, protein, and fertility-boosting nutrients.

<u>Prep Time</u>: 20 minutes

14. Beef and Vegetable Stir-Fry

<u>Ingredients</u>:

1 lb lean beef strips

Broccoli florets

Snow peas

Bell peppers, sliced

Garlic, minced

Soy sauce

Sesame oil

<u>Preparation</u>:

Stir-fry beef in sesame oil until browned.

Add garlic, broccoli, snow peas, and bell peppers. Cook until veggies are tender.

Pour in soy sauce and toss until everything is well-coated.

<u>Nutritional Value</u>: High in protein, iron, and fertility-boosting nutrients.

<u>Prep Time</u>: 25 minutes

15. Quinoa and Sweet Potato Buddha Bowl

<u>Ingredients</u>:

1 cup quinoa

2 sweet potatoes, diced

Chickpeas, drained

Kale leaves

Tahini dressing

Lemon wedges

<u>Preparation</u>:

Cook quinoa according to package instructions.

Roast sweet potatoes and chickpeas in olive oil until crispy.

Assemble bowls with quinoa, roasted sweet potatoes, chickpeas, and kale.

Serve with lemon wedges and a drizzle of tahini dressing.

<u>Nutritional Value</u>: Packed with antioxidants, fiber, and fertility-boosting nutrients.

<u>Prep Time</u>: 35 minutes

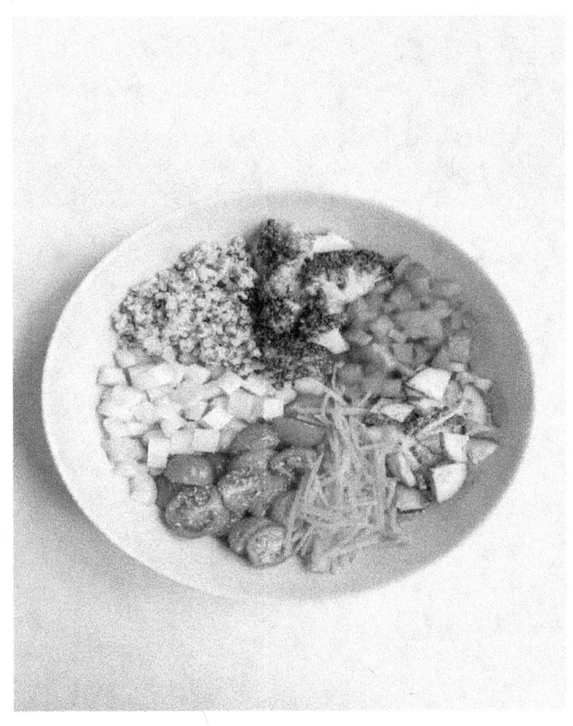

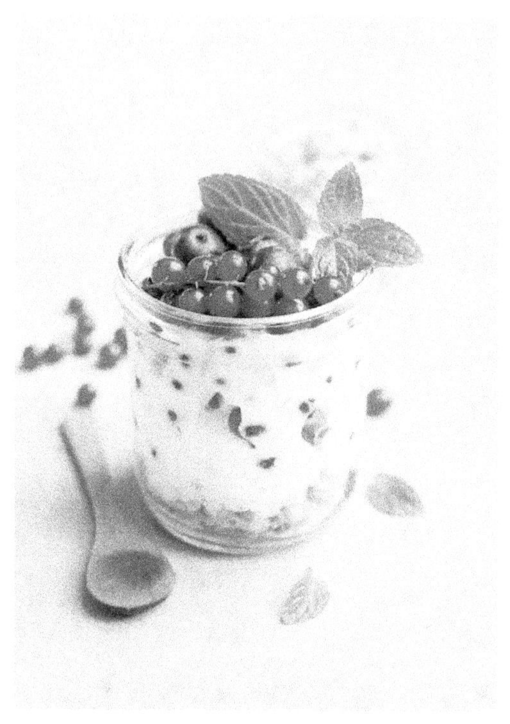

Chapter 6

SNACKS AND TREATS

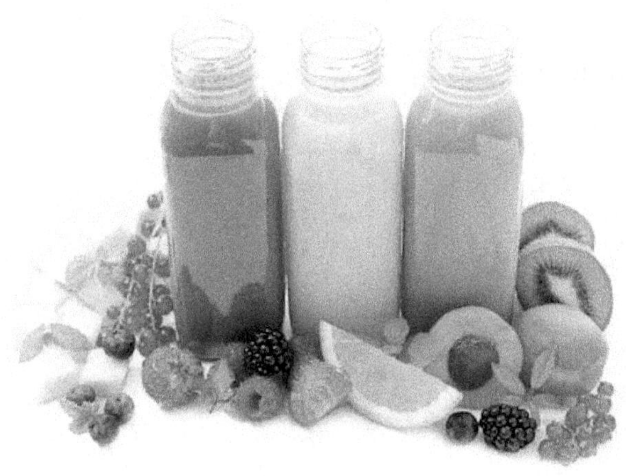

1. Berry Bliss Smoothie Bowl

<u>Ingredients:</u>

1 cup mixed berries (strawberries, blueberries, raspberries)

1 banana, frozen

1/2 cup Greek yogurt

1 tablespoon honey

<u>Preparation:</u>

Blend berries, banana, and yogurt until smooth.

Pour into a bowl, drizzle with honey.

<u>Nutritional Value:</u> High in antioxidants, vitamins, and probiotics.

<u>Prep Time:</u> 5 minutes

2. Avocado and Tomato Bruschetta

<u>Ingredients:</u>

2 ripe avocados, mashed

1 cup cherry tomatoes, diced

2 tablespoons olive oil

1 clove garlic, minced

<u>Preparation:</u>

Spread crushed avocado mixture onto each slice of toast, then generously spoon tomato topping on top. Add basil as a garnish and serve right away.

<u>Nutritional Value:</u> Healthy fats, vitamins, and minerals.

<u>Prep Time</u>: 10 minutes

3. Quinoa and Spinach Patties

<u>Ingredients:</u>

1 cup cooked quinoa

1 cup chopped spinach

1/4 cup feta cheese, crumbled

1 egg

<u>Preparation:</u>

Mix cooked quinoa, spinach, feta, and egg.

Form into patties and cook until golden.

<u>Nutritional Value</u>: Protein, iron, and folate.

<u>Prep Time</u>: 15 minutes

4. Chia Seed Pudding

<u>Ingredients:</u>

3 tablespoons chia seeds

1 cup almond milk

1 teaspoon vanilla extract

Fresh berries for topping

<u>Preparation</u>:

Mix chia seeds, almond milk, and vanilla. Refrigerate.

Top with fresh berries before serving.

<u>Nutritional Value</u>: Omega-3 fatty acids, fiber, and calcium.

<u>Prep Time</u>: 5 minutes (+ refrigeration time)

5. Sweet Potato and Chickpea Bites

<u>Ingredients</u>:

1 cup sweet potato, grated

1 can chickpeas, drained

2 tablespoons olive oil

1 teaspoon cumin

<u>Preparation</u>:

Blend sweet potato, chickpeas, olive oil, and cumin.

Form into small bites and bake.

<u>Nutritional Value</u>: Fiber, vitamins, and protein.

<u>Prep Time</u>: 20 minutes

6. Edamame and Almond Trail Mix

<u>Ingredients</u>:

1 cup edamame, steamed

1/2 cup almonds

1/4 cup dried cranberries

1 teaspoon sea salt

<u>Preparation</u>:

Mix edamame, almonds, and cranberries.

Sprinkle with sea salt.

<u>Nutritional Value</u>: Protein, fiber, and antioxidants.

<u>Prep Time</u>: 5 minutes

7. Pineapple and Ginger Smoothie

<u>Ingredients</u>:

1 cup pineapple chunks

1 inch fresh ginger, grated

1/2 cup coconut milk

1 tablespoon flaxseeds

Preparation:

Blend pineapple, ginger, coconut milk, and flaxseeds.

Serve over ice.

<u>Nutritional Value</u>: Bromelain, anti-inflammatory properties, and omega-3s.

<u>Prep Time</u>: 8 minutes

8. Mango and Avocado Salsa

<u>Ingredients</u>:

1 ripe mango, diced

1 avocado, diced

1/2 red onion, finely chopped

1 lime, juiced

<u>Preparation</u>:

Mix mango, avocado, red onion, and lime juice.

Chill before serving with whole-grain chips.

<u>Nutritional Value</u>: Vitamins, healthy fats, and antioxidants.

<u>Prep Time</u>: 12 minutes

9. Cottage Cheese and Pineapple Parfait

<u>Ingredients</u>:

1 cup low-fat cottage cheese

1 cup fresh pineapple chunks

1/4 cup granola

1 tablespoon honey

<u>Preparation</u>:

Layer cottage cheese, pineapple, and granola.

Drizzle with honey.

<u>Nutritional Value</u>: Protein, vitamin C, and probiotics.

<u>Prep Time</u>: 5 minutes

10. Spinach and Feta Stuffed Mushrooms

<u>Ingredients</u>:

12 large mushrooms, stems removed

1 cup spinach, chopped

1/2 cup feta cheese, crumbled

1 tablespoon olive oil

<u>Preparation</u>:

Saute spinach in olive oil, mix with feta.

Stuff mushrooms and bake.

<u>Nutritional Value</u>: Iron, folate, and calcium.

<u>Prep Time</u>: 25 minutes

11. Walnut and Banana Muffins

<u>Ingredients:</u>

1 cup whole wheat flour

1/2 cup chopped walnuts

2 ripe bananas, mashed

1/4 cup honey

<u>Preparation:</u>

Mix flour, walnuts, mashed bananas, and honey.

Bake into muffins.

<u>Nutritional Value</u>: Omega-3s, fiber, and potassium.

<u>Prep Time</u>: 18 minutes

12. Caprese Salad Skewers

<u>Ingredients:</u>

Cherry tomatoes

Fresh mozzarella balls

Basil leaves

Balsamic glaze

<u>Preparation</u>:

Skewer tomatoes, mozzarella, and basil.

Drizzle with balsamic glaze.

<u>Nutritional Value</u>: Calcium, antioxidants, and vitamins.

<u>Prep Time</u>: 10 minutes

13. Almond Butter and Banana Sandwich

<u>Ingredients</u>:

4 slices whole-grain bread

2 tablespoons almond butter

1 banana, sliced

Cinnamon (optional)

<u>Preparation</u>:

Spread almond butter on bread, add banana slices.

Sprinkle with cinnamon if desired.

<u>Nutritional Value</u>: Protein, potassium, and healthy fats.

<u>Prep Time</u>: 5 minutes

14. Roasted Red Pepper Hummus Dip

<u>Ingredients</u>:

1 can chickpeas, drained

1/4 cup tahini

1/4 cup roasted red peppers

2 cloves garlic

<u>Preparation</u>:

Blend chickpeas, tahini, red peppers, and garlic.

Serve with carrot and cucumber sticks.

<u>Nutritional Value</u>: Protein, fiber, and vitamins.

15. Chocolate Avocado Mousse

Ingredients:

2 ripe avocados

1/4 cup cocoa powder

1/4 cup maple syrup

1 teaspoon vanilla extract

Preparation:

Blend avocados, cocoa powder, maple syrup, and vanilla.

Refrigerate before serving.

Nutritional Value: Healthy fats, antioxidants, and minerals.

Prep Time: 10 minutes

Chapter 7

BEVERAGES

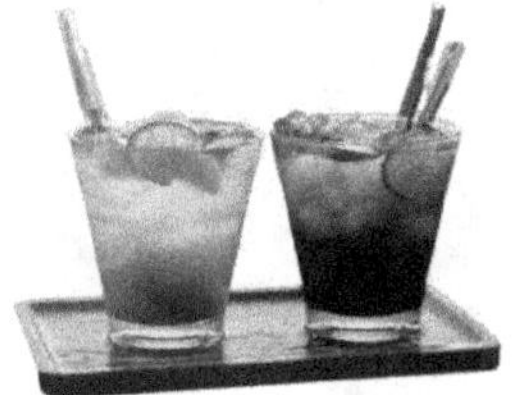

1. Green Fertility Smoothie

Ingredients:

1 cup spinach leaves

1/2 avocado

1/2 cup pineapple chunks

1 cup almond milk

Nutritional Value: Rich in folate and vitamin C

<u>Preparation:</u>

Blend all ingredients until smooth.

<u>Prep Time:</u> 5 minutes

2. Berry Blast Fertility Juice

<u>Ingredients:</u>

1 cup mixed berries (strawberries, blueberries, raspberries)

1/2 cup Greek yogurt

1 tablespoon honey

1 cup coconut water

<u>Nutritional Value:</u> Antioxidants and probiotics

<u>Preparation:</u>

Blend berries, yogurt, honey, and coconut water.

<u>Prep Time:</u> 7 minutes

3. Pomegranate Citrus Elixir

<u>Ingredients</u>:

1/2 cup pomegranate seeds

Juice of 1 orange

1 teaspoon chia seeds

1 cup water

<u>Nutritional Value</u>: High in antioxidants and omega-3 fatty acids

Preparation:

Mix all ingredients and let sit for 10 minutes before consuming.

<u>Prep Time:</u> 2 minutes

4. Turmeric Spice Infusion

<u>Ingredients</u>:

1 teaspoon turmeric powder

1/2 teaspoon ginger, grated

1 tablespoon honey

1 cup warm water

Nutritional Value: Anti-inflammatory properties

Preparation: Mix turmeric, ginger, and honey in warm water.

Prep Time: 3 minutes

5. Protein-Packed Almond Shake

Ingredients:

1 scoop fertility-friendly protein powder

1 cup almond milk

1/2 banana

1 tablespoon flaxseeds

Nutritional Value: High protein and omega-3 fatty acids

Preparation:

Blend protein powder, almond milk, banana, and flaxseeds.

Prep Time: 5 minutes

6. Ginger Lemonade Cooler

<u>Ingredients</u>:

1 tablespoon fresh ginger, grated

Juice of 2 lemons

1 tablespoon maple syrup

2 cups cold water

<u>Nutritional Value</u>: Supports digestion and vitamin C

<u>Preparation</u>:

Mix ginger, lemon juice, maple syrup, and cold water.

<u>Prep Time</u>: 5 minutes

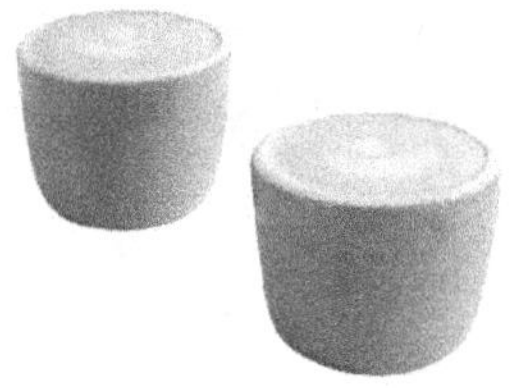

7. Chia Seed Hydration

Ingredients:

2 tablespoons chia seeds

1 cup coconut water

1/2 cup mango chunks

Nutritional Value: Omega-3 fatty acids and hydration

Preparation:

Combine chia seeds, coconut water, and mango. Stir well and let sit for 15 minutes.

Prep Time: 17 minutes (including soaking time)

8. Cucumber Mint Refresher

Ingredients:

1/2 cucumber, sliced

Handful of mint leaves

1 tablespoon honey

2 cups water

<u>Nutritional Value</u>: Hydration and soothing properties

<u>Preparation</u>:

Mix cucumber, mint, honey, and water. Give the flavours 30 minutes to fully meld.

<u>Prep Time</u>: 30 minutes

9. Folate-Rich Carrot Juice

<u>Ingredients</u>:

4 medium carrots, juiced

1/2 orange, juiced

1 tablespoon ginger, grated

<u>Nutritional Value:</u> High in folate and vitamin A

<u>Preparation</u>:

Juice carrots and orange, then add grated ginger.

<u>Prep Time</u>: 5 minutes

10. Cocoa Banana Smoothie

Ingredients:

2 tablespoons cocoa powder

1 cup almond milk

1 large banana

1 tablespoon peanut butter

Nutritional Value: Rich in antioxidants and potassium

Preparation:

Blend cocoa powder, almond milk, banana, and peanut butter.

Prep Time: 4 minutes

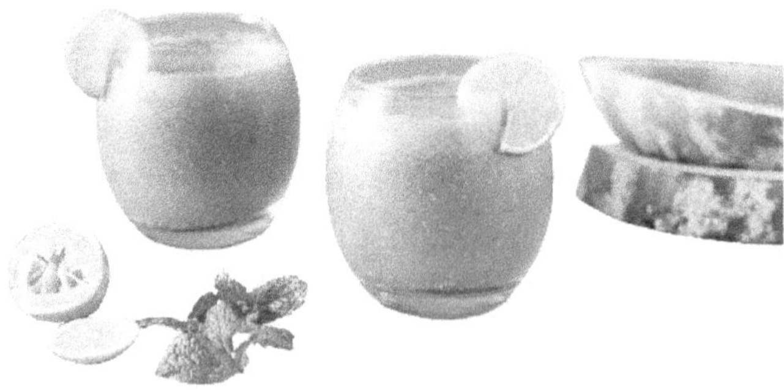

11. Spinach and Pineapple Detox

Ingredients:

2 cups spinach leaves

1 cup pineapple chunks

1/2 lemon, juiced

1 cup coconut water

Nutritional Value: Detoxifying and vitamin C

Preparation:

Blend spinach, pineapple, lemon juice, and coconut water.

Prep Time: 6 minutes

12. Hibiscus Berry Tea

Ingredients:

2 hibiscus tea bags

1/2 cup mixed berries

1 tablespoon honey

2 cups hot water

Nutritional Value: Antioxidants and immune support

Preparation:

Steep hibiscus tea bags in hot water, then add berries and honey.

Prep Time: 8 minutes

13. Mango Lassi

Ingredients:

1 cup plain Greek yogurt

1/2 cup mango chunks

1 tablespoon honey

1/2 teaspoon cardamom

Nutritional Value: Probiotics and vitamin C

Preparation:

Blend yogurt, mango, honey, and cardamom until smooth.

Prep Time: 5 minutes

14. Beetroot Berry Elixir

Ingredients:

1/2 medium beetroot, juiced

1/2 cup mixed berries

1 tablespoon chia seeds

Nutritional Value: Rich in antioxidants and iron

Preparation:

Mix beetroot juice, mixed berries, and chia seeds.

Prep Time: 3 minutes

15. Lemon Ginger Green Tea

Ingredients:

2 green tea bags

1 tablespoon fresh ginger, grated

Juice of 1 lemon

2 cups hot water

<u>Nutritional Value:</u> Antioxidants and digestive support

<u>Preparation:</u>

Steep green tea bags in hot water, then add ginger and lemon juice.

<u>Prep Time:</u> 5 minutes

Chapter 8

LIFESTYLE PRACTICES FOR FERTILITY

Incorporating Exercise into Your Routine

Does physical exercise interfere with getting pregnant?

"Can I exercise while trying to get pregnant?" is a common question that women have been asking when they decide to try for a baby

Pregnancy is a beautiful moment in women's lives, but it can also be a process full of doubts. With so much information available about fertility, it's easy to feel confused and not know what to really believe. One of the questions that many women ask themselves is whether physical exercise interferes with getting pregnant.

But, can exercising really harm fertility? Or does it actually help to have a baby?

The relationship between physical exercise and female fertility is full of questions and depends on several factors. Keep reading!

The practice of physical exercise and fertility

Fertility can be affected for a variety of reasons, including age, lifestyle, stress , polycystic ovary syndrome (PCOS) , body weight, among others. There is some information that reports on the impact of physical exercise on women's fertility. However, it is worth highlighting that this is not absolutely true!

In general, practicing physical activity has many benefits for female reproductive health. Some studies indicate that exercising regularly helps reduce conditions that affect the pregnancy process, such as diabetes, obesity and PCOS.

Other advantages of physical exercise are: reducing stress, improving mood and controlling weight. The latter, for example, indicates that if a woman has a healthy body mass index (BMI), consequently, she has a greater chance of getting pregnant. Therefore, it is essential to have an exercise routine to maintain your ideal weight and improve your chances of having a baby.

High intensity activities

There are some types of exercises that are more intense and have negative impacts. For example, long-distance running and weight lifting can increase levels of cortisol, which is the stress hormone, and thus affect ovulation. Resistance training is likely to cause hormonal imbalance or even a reduction in estrogen.

Furthermore, if you do not have adequate guidance from a physical education and nutrition professional, high intensity exercise can lead to excessive weight loss, damaging fertility.

If you are a woman who is already accustomed to high-intensity physical exercise, but who wants to get pregnant, it is worth seeking out a fertility specialist to obtain all the necessary information on the subject.

It is possible to adapt your training routine, but in a way that does not harm the pregnancy process.

Low intensity activities

On the other hand, activities that do not require as much intensity, such as walking, for example, do not have a negative impact on fertility. In fact, it is highly recommended to carry out this type of activity on a daily basis, as it improves blood circulation and also reduces stress levels.

Another factor is that light physical exercise does not cause excessive weight loss, unlike what we mentioned in the previous topic.

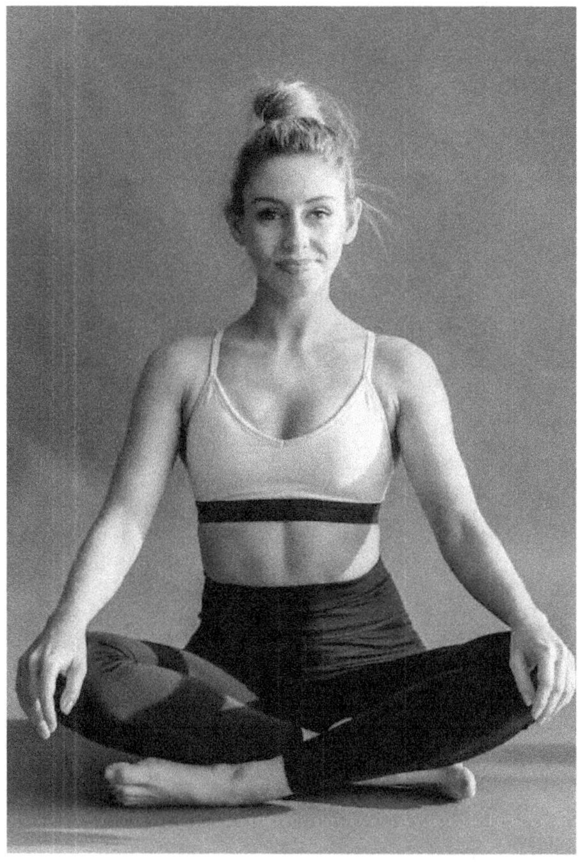

3 physical exercises that help with fertility

So far we have seen that physical exercise has its peculiarities in relation to fertility. It is worth highlighting that the interference of the practice depends from woman to woman, mainly due to their lifestyle and health history.

1. Walk

It is a low-impact exercise that can be easily incorporated into your daily routine, without the need to go to gyms or even purchase special equipment.

You will only need willingness, light clothing and good walking shoes. After that, set aside 30 minutes a day, three to five times a week, to move your body.

2. Pilates

Pilates is also another recommended physical exercise for fertility. It helps to strengthen the body, especially the abdominal and lower back muscles, and also to improve posture.

Furthermore, activity helps to increase flexibility and reduce stress, which are beneficial factors for reproductive health.

3. Yoga

It is an activity that combines breathing and meditation techniques, which are essential for reducing anxiety and stress. Additionally, yoga helps improve muscle strengthening and flexibility.

As we have seen, physical exercise has positive impacts, but is prone to negative consequences on female fertility. Therefore, it is essential to be careful with the intensity of training.

What are the benefits of physical activities for those who want to get pregnant?

The benefits of practicing physical exercise daily are immense and extremely important for anyone's health. However, if the desire to become pregnant is present, this action increases its importance even more.

Discover 5 important reasons for physical activity during pregnancy;

1. Increased fertility

Practicing moderate-intensity physical activity can significantly increase fertility. If the exercises are done in a regular and balanced way, the female body will find itself increasingly healthier for pregnancy. This is done by maintaining the ideal weight and the correct functioning of the metabolism.

The recommendation, along with a moderate exercise routine, is to follow a healthy diet because it is important to have a minimum amount of body fat to get pregnant. For men, regular exercise can also improve sperm quality.

On the other hand, it will be difficult to get pregnant if the physical exercises chosen are exaggerated or high-impact, as well as if the woman does not exercise significantly.

2. Stimulation of improvement of the cardiovascular and respiratory system

Pregnancy demands a lot of health from the female body, which increases the need to be well aligned, mainly with the cardiovascular and respiratory systems. At the beginning of pregnancy, it is essential that these body functions meet the increased demands of the mother's body.

Furthermore, as the baby grows, the space inside the mother ends up pushing on some organs, such as the lungs. Therefore, if the woman has already been practicing light physical exercise before pregnancy, this discomfort and the resulting tiredness may decrease.

3. Adapting to body change

The increase in the volume of the uterus , abdominal region and breasts alters the female gravitational center, causing greater discomfort in supporting the body, especially in the first months of pregnancy. Therefore, active women adapt much better to the new gravitational center than sedentary women.

Likewise, women who exercise regularly are able to relax, reducing stress and possible bouts of insomnia . Furthermore, muscle and bone discomfort, caused by the growth of the fetus, is reduced.

4. Preventing overweight

Women who exercise before becoming pregnant avoid the unwanted excess weight that appears during pregnancy. Therefore, in addition to reducing body fat levels, practicing physical activity facilitates weight loss after childbirth.

5. Strengthening muscles

Physical exercises help to strengthen certain muscles that are important for women seeking a natural birth. They are;

- ❖ lower back : needs to be strong to avoid severe back pain , which is caused by muscles not prepared for pregnancy;
- ❖ pelvic floor: important to generate more strength for normal birth and help with constant trips to the bathroom at the end of pregnancy.

Pay attention to exercises

It is important that the exercises are consistent for six months prior to fertilization. Therefore, the ideal is to opt for light exercises , such as walking and water aerobics , for example. If you want to get pregnant, pay attention to these tips to prepare for your baby's arrival.

The Role of Sleep in Fertility

Sleep plays a crucial role in overall health and well-being, and it can significantly impact fertility for both men and women. Here are several ways in which sleep influences fertility:

- Hormonal Balance:

Adequate sleep is essential for maintaining hormonal balance. Sleep deprivation can disrupt the production of hormones such as cortisol, insulin, and reproductive hormones like luteinizing hormone (LH) and follicle-stimulating hormone (FSH).

These hormonal disruptions can affect menstrual cycles in women and sperm production in men.

- Menstrual Regularity:

Women with irregular sleep patterns or insufficient sleep may experience irregular menstrual cycles or disruptions in ovulation.

Consistent sleeping patterns help regulate the body's internal clock, which is crucial for maintaining a regular menstrual cycle.

- Testosterone Levels in Men:

In men, testosterone is essential for sperm production. Sleep deprivation or poor sleep quality can lead to a decline in testosterone levels.

Lower testosterone levels may negatively impact sperm quality and fertility.

- Ovulation and Egg Quality:

Adequate sleep contributes to the proper regulation of the menstrual cycle and ovulation.

Quality sleep is associated with better egg quality, which is crucial for successful conception.

- Stress Reduction:

Sleep is a key factor in stress management. Chronic stress can negatively affect fertility by disrupting hormonal balance.

Quality sleep helps the body recover from daily stressors and promotes emotional well-being.

- Immune System Function:

Sleep is essential for a well-functioning immune system. A strong immune system is crucial for a healthy pregnancy.

Inadequate sleep can compromise the immune system, making the body more susceptible to infections that might impact fertility.

- Sperm Health:

Sufficient sleep is associated with better sperm health. Men who consistently get an adequate amount of sleep tend to have higher sperm counts and better sperm motility.

Poor sleep quality or sleep disorders may contribute to male infertility.

- Optimal Body Weight:

Sleep influences metabolic processes, and inadequate sleep has been linked to weight gain and obesity.

Maintaining a healthy body weight is important for fertility, as both underweight and overweight conditions can impact reproductive function.

To promote fertility through better sleep:

- Aim for 7-9 hours of quality sleep per night.
- Ensure you have a consistent sleep hour that spans throughout the week

- Create a sleep-conducive environment by keeping the bedroom dark, quiet, and cool.

- Limit screen time before bedtime to improve the quality of sleep.

If fertility issues persist, consulting with a healthcare professional specializing in reproductive health can provide additional insights and guidance tailored to individual circumstances

Stress Management Techniques for Both Partners

Stress can have a significant impact on fertility for both partners. High stress levels can affect hormonal balance, disrupt menstrual cycles, and reduce sperm production. Implementing stress management techniques can be beneficial for improving fertility. Here are some techniques that both partners can consider:

- Mindfulness Meditation:

To reduce stress and promote a sense of calm, engage in mindfulness meditation

Couples can practice mindfulness together or individually for a few minutes each day.

- Deep Breathing Exercises:

Deep breathing exercises can activate the relaxation response and reduce stress.

Practice deep, slow breaths to calm the nervous system and promote relaxation.

- Regular Exercise:

Engaging in regular physical activity can help reduce stress and improve overall well-being.

Choose activities that you both enjoy, such as walking, yoga, or dancing.

- Healthy Lifestyle Choices:

Maintain a balanced diet, ensure you take adequate nutrients that are essential.

Limit caffeine and alcohol intake, as they can contribute to stress and fertility issues.

- Open Communication:

Foster open communication between partners to share concerns, fears, and emotions.

Discussing feelings can strengthen the emotional connection and reduce stress.

- Couples Counseling

Seeking professional help can provide a safe space for couples to explore and address underlying stressors.

A counselor can offer guidance on coping strategies and communication skills.

- Relaxation Techniques:

Engage in relaxation techniques such as progressive muscle relaxation or exercise. These techniques can help ease tension and create a more relaxed state of mind.

- Prioritize Sleep:

Ensure both partners are getting sufficient and quality sleep.

Lack of sleep can contribute to stress, so establishing good sleep hygiene is crucial.

- Time Management:

Create a realistic schedule that allows for work, relaxation, and quality time together.

Prioritize activities that bring joy and relaxation.

- Acupuncture and Massage

Some couples find acupuncture or massage therapy beneficial for stress reduction. Consult with healthcare professionals to explore these complementary therapies.

- Hobbies and Leisure Activities:

Engage in activities that bring joy and relaxation, whether it's reading, gardening, or pursuing hobbies together.

It's important to remember that fertility issues can be complex, and stress is just one factor. If difficulties persist, seeking guidance from healthcare professionals specializing in fertility can be beneficial. They can provide personalized advice based on the specific needs and circumstances of the couple.

Chapter 9

BONUS (FREE 15 SMOOTHIES)

Here's the bonus for you, 15 smoothies recipes.+

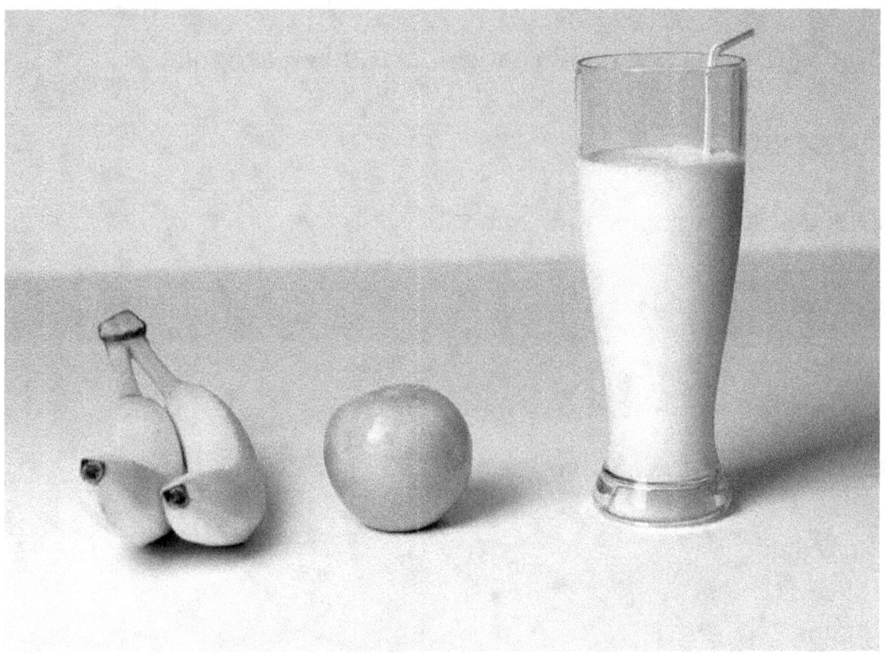

1. Berry Boost Smoothie

<u>Ingredients:</u>

1 cup mixed berries (strawberries, blueberries, raspberries)

1 banana

1/2 cup Greek yogurt

1 tablespoon chia seeds

1 cup spinach

1 cup almond milk

Nutritional Value: High in antioxidants, fiber, and folate.

Preparation:

Blend all ingredients until smooth.

Serve immediately.

2. Green Goddess Smoothie

Ingredients:

2 cups kale

1/2 cucumber

1/2 avocado

1 kiwi, peeled

1 tablespoon flaxseeds

1 cup coconut water

Nutritional Value: Rich in folate, vitamin C, and healthy fats.

Preparation:

Blend all ingredients until creamy.

Pour into glasses and enjoy.

3. Pineapple Passion Smoothie

Ingredients:

1 cup pineapple chunks

1/2 mango

1/2 cup carrots, grated

1 tablespoon pumpkin seeds

1 cup coconut milk

Nutritional Value: Contains bromelain, vitamin A, and zinc.

Preparation:

Blend until smooth and pour into glasses.

4. Citrus Delight Smoothie

<u>Ingredients:</u>

2 oranges, peeled

1 cup strawberries

1/2 cup Greek yogurt

1 tablespoon hemp seeds

1 cup water

<u>Nutritional Value:</u> High in vitamin C, antioxidants, and protein.

<u>Preparation:</u>

In a blender, combine all the ingredients and blend till smooth

5. Banana Berry Bliss Smoothie

<u>Ingredients:</u>

2 bananas

1 cup mixed berries (blueberries, raspberries)

1/2 cup spinach

1 tablespoon almond butter

1 cup almond milk

<u>Nutritional Value:</u> Packed with potassium, antioxidants, and iron.

<u>Preparation:</u>

Blend until creamy and pour into glasses.

6. Mango Tango Fertility Smoothie

<u>Ingredients:</u>

1 cup mango chunks

1/2 cup pineapple

1/2 cup Greek yogurt

1 tablespoon chia seeds

1 cup coconut water

<u>Nutritional Value:</u> Rich in vitamin E, zinc, and probiotics.

<u>Preparation:</u>

Blend until smooth and enjoy immediately.

7. Avocado Almond Joy Smoothie

Ingredients:

1/2 avocado

1/4 cup almonds

1 tablespoon cacao powder

1 tablespoon honey

1 cup almond milk

Nutritional Value: Good source of healthy fats, vitamin E, and magnesium.

Preparation:

Blend until creamy and serve.

8. Blueberry Spinach Power Smoothie

Ingredients:

1 cup blueberries

1 cup spinach

1/2 cup plain yogurt

1 tablespoon flaxseeds

1 cup water

<u>Nutritional Value:</u> High in antioxidants, iron, and probiotics.

<u>Preparation:</u>

Blend all ingredients until smooth and enjoy.

9. Strawberry Kiwi Quencher

<u>Ingredients:</u>

1 cup strawberries

2 kiwis, peeled

1/2 cup coconut water

1 tablespoon chia seeds

1 cup ice cubes

<u>Nutritional Value:</u> High in vitamin C, fibre, and omega-3 fatty acids.

<u>Preparation:</u>

Blend until slushy and pour into glasses.

10. Cherry Chocolate Smoothie

Ingredients:

1 cup cherries, pitted

1/2 banana

2 tablespoons dark chocolate chips

1 tablespoon almond butter

1 cup almond milk

Nutritional Value: Contains antioxidants, potassium, and healthy fats.

Preparation:

Blend until smooth and top with a few extra cherries if desired.

11. Pomegranate Paradise Smoothie

Ingredients:

1 cup pomegranate seeds

1/2 cup raspberries

1/2 cup plain yogurt

1 tablespoon pumpkin seeds

1 cup water

Nutritional Value: High in antioxidants, vitamin K, and protein.

Preparation:

Blend until creamy and pour into glasses.

12. Almond Joyful Fertility Smoothie

Ingredients:

1/4 cup almonds

1/2 banana

1 tablespoon cacao powder

1 tablespoon almond butter

1 cup coconut milk

Nutritional Value: Good source of healthy fats, magnesium, and iron.

Preparation:

Blend until smooth and enjoy.

13. Raspberry Oatmeal Elixir

<u>Ingredients:</u>

1 cup raspberries

1/2 cup oats

1/2 cup plain yogurt

1 tablespoon honey

1 cup almond milk

<u>Nutritional Value:</u> Rich in fiber, protein, and antioxidants.

<u>Preparation:</u>

Blend until creamy and serve immediately.

14. Cacao Banana Berry Blend

<u>Ingredients:</u>

1/2 cup mixed berries (strawberries, blueberries)

1 banana

1 tablespoon cacao powder

1 tablespoon almond butter

1 cup coconut water

Nutritional Value: Contains antioxidants, potassium, and healthy fats.

Preparation:

Blend until smooth and pour into glasses.

15. Spinach Mango Tango

Ingredients:

2 cups spinach

1 cup mango chunks

1/2 banana

1 tablespoon chia seeds

1 cup water

Nutritional Value: High in vitamin A, iron, and omega-3 fatty acids.

Preparation:

Blend until creamy and enjoy immediately.

Conclusion

In conclusion, this fertility diet cookbook is not just a collection of recipes but a holistic guide to nourishing your body for optimal reproductive health. Through careful consideration of nutrient-dense ingredients and mindful culinary choices, this cookbook aims to empower you on your journey towards enhanced fertility.

I've explored the science behind fertility-boosting foods, delving into the vital role that nutrition plays in reproductive wellness. From fertility-friendly nutrients like folate, zinc, and antioxidants to the importance of maintaining a healthy weight, the recipes presented here are crafted to support your reproductive system at every stage.

Moreover, the culinary journey embarked upon in this cookbook is not just about achieving a short-term goal but fostering a lifestyle that promotes lasting well-being. By incorporating these delicious and nutritious recipes into your daily routine, you're not only optimizing your chances of conception but also embracing a path towards overall health and vitality.

As you embark on this culinary adventure, remember that the choices you make in the kitchen have the power to influence not only your fertility but your entire well-being. So, let this cookbook serve as a guide to not just meals, but to a lifestyle that harmonizes nutrition, fertility, and overall health.

In adopting and adapting to this fertility diet, envision the incredible potential within yourself to create a nurturing environment for new beginnings.

Your journey towards fertility is a personal narrative, and this cookbook is a tool to help you script a story of resilience, health, and joy. Embrace the nourishing power of these recipes, and let your culinary choices be a celebration of life and the limitless possibilities it holds.